Overcoming Co

Stammering
Advice for all ages

RENÉE BYRNE AND LOUISE WRIGHT

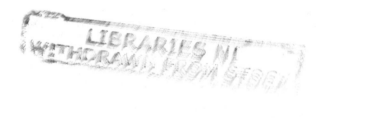
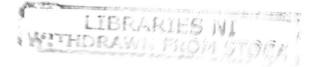
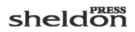

sheldon PRESS

*This book is dedicated to all our clients, colleagues and friends
who stammer, especially those who contributed their stories to
the final chapter of the book*

First published in Great Britain in 2008

Sheldon Press
36 Causton Street
London SW1P 4ST

British Library Cataloguing-in-Publication Data
A catalogue record for this book is available from the British Library

ISBN 978–1–84709–020–1

1 3 5 7 9 10 8 6 4 2

Typeset by Fakenham Photosetting Ltd, Fakenham, Norfolk
Printed in Great Britain by Ashford Colour Press

Produced on paper from sustainable forests

Contents

Acknowledgements

With thanks to Fiona Marshall of Sheldon Press for her guidance and encouragement. Special thanks to our husbands, Peter Byrne and Keith Busby, for help with the manuscript and illustrations respectively, but most importantly for their love and support in a challenging year.

Preface

About the book

This book is written for everyone who stammers, and for parents, teachers, friends and all those concerned with, or interested in, this subject. The authors are speech and language therapists with considerable practical experience of working with children and adults who stammer, as well as having academic knowledge from their work as university lecturers. This is not a technical book – there are many of those on the market. Our aim is to offer jargon-free information and treatment guidelines about stammering, from childhood to maturity.

Explanation

You will see from the contents page that we move from childhood through to the teenage years and then on to adulthood. There are significant differences in the speech and the treatment at various stages, but there are also certain similarities. The best way of using this book is to read it from the beginning, regardless of the particular age group that interests you. In this way you get an overview of this somewhat complicated subject, and you may find it interesting to see how stammering develops – or how it is arrested. Our chapters are roughly divided into those concerned with children, then teenagers, followed by adults, because that seems the obvious progression. Chronologically, these are distinct age groups but, in the real world, there is no definite age when a child matures into a teenager or a teenager becomes an adult.

The words we use

We have used the word 'stammer' because it is recognized in many parts of the world and, although 'stutter' is often heard both in the UK and elsewhere, 'stammer' is generally acceptable.

When using the term 'therapist', we are referring to registered speech and language therapists. This in no way implies that we are negating the work of other professionals and alternative practitioners offering a variety of conventional and unconventional treatment approaches.

We hope that no confusion will be caused by our use of the abbreviation SLT for speech and language therapist, as well as for speech and language therapy.

Stammerer, the person who stammers (PWS)

Some people feel quite strongly about the words used to describe someone with a stammer. In the past, 'stammerer' was the accepted term, but in recent years 'people who stammer' has come into the vocabulary because it was thought that using the term 'stammerer' defines a person purely by one characteristic and, obviously, there is much more to people than the way they speak. Some books are now using the abbreviation PWS ('Person Who Stammers'), but neither the authors of this book, nor their clients, like that acronym. We have decided to use 'stammerer' and 'person who stammers' – the former because it is less clumsy when written and the latter to remind us all – those who stammer, their families, friends, therapists and everyone interested in the subject – that the stammer is only one part of a child, a teenager or an adult.

Names used

When quoting clients or writing case studies, all names have been changed to ensure anonymity – with the exception of Chapter 13, where many of the contributors have chosen to use their own names.

Acquired stammering

The sudden onset of stammering caused by a head injury or some other medical or psychological condition is not within the scope of this book.

1

An introduction to stammering

'Stuttering' and 'stammering' are two words that mean the same thing. In the UK, 'stammering' is probably the most familiar word but, because some other English-speaking countries use 'stuttering', both words are creeping into the UK vocabulary. The important point is that there is no difference – both words mean:

Speech that is hesitant, stumbling, tense or jerky so that the smooth flow is interrupted.

That aspect of stammering – the speech part – is known to most of us and is fairly obvious, but there is another less obvious and frequently hidden part. Before explaining that statement, we need to clarify a fundamental issue.

If you are reading this book because you are concerned about the speech of a young child, then it is most important that you understand that there is a crucial difference between beginning stammering and the confirmed condition. The difference is that, while early stammering in young children is largely a temporary speech difficulty, for some older children and all adults, the condition is more than that – more than solely a speech condition.

People who stammer know exactly what they want to say but, at that moment, they are unable to say it easily, and this causes a variety of feelings and emotions such as frustration, anger, embarrassment and anxiety to develop and grow over the years. These feelings and emotions about their stammer, and about themselves as people who stammer, become an integral part of the confirmed situation.

Stammering is not just one condition – it covers a range of difficulties from severe to mild and, because it is essentially a developmental condition, it changes over time. The following examples demonstrate this:

Colin, 4, was brought to the speech and language therapy clinic by his mother because she had become concerned about the constant repetitions in his speech. Colin was certainly showing marked signs of early stammering, but our observations, and his mother's report, indicated that he was a chatty little boy and unconcerned about his speech difficulty.

Mala, 15, attended the clinic and stated that she stammered a lot and felt that she was only fluent perhaps 40 per cent of the time, but that she was always completely fluent when talking to her mother and to her best friend. She was worried about her stammer because she was afraid to speak out at school, and was now facing choices about careers.

Josh, 28, came to therapy a few weeks after Mala, saying that he hardly stammered at all, and that he was fluent perhaps 90 per cent of the time. He came for advice because, whenever he had to speak to someone in authority at work, certain words somehow got stuck. He used the phone as little as possible and was thinking of turning down a promotion because it involved giving presentations, and no one at work knew he stammered.

An essential factor is the developmental nature of this condition, such that Colin's symptoms may seem quite severe but, at his age, he could definitely still become a fluent speaker. Moreover, he has not as yet acquired a range of negative feelings about the way that he speaks.

Mala and Josh are at a different stage of development because although for Mala there is a slight possibility of recovery, Josh is certainly in the confirmed stage of stammering and there is a distinct possibility that his is an on-going difficulty.

Why is stammering like an iceberg?

It has proved helpful to discuss stammering in terms of an iceberg because, using this analogy,[1] we can explain three important aspects:

- The development of stammering from childhood.
- The individual nature of the condition.
- The variability of treatment approaches.

One part of an iceberg can be clearly seen above the surface of the water, but another, and sometimes more significant, part is hidden below the water. Although concealed, this part is an integral component of the iceberg. Stammering can be compared to an iceberg because the part above the surface, the speech, can be heard and seen (overt); the feelings and attitudes, which have not formed in early childhood, but are a crucial aspect of confirmed stammering, are the hidden part held inside the speaker and unknown to the listener (covert).

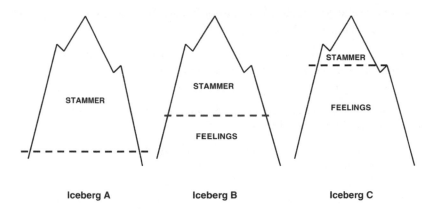

Figure 1.1   The stammering 'icebergs'

When you look at these representations of the stammering 'icebergs' (Figure 1.1), it is clear that the overt and covert elements differ markedly between the three 'icebergs'.

In iceberg A, there is a speech difficulty with few, if any, feelings associated with speaking – perhaps a child such as Colin, mentioned above.

In iceberg B, the speaker has roughly a 50:50 ratio situation where the stammer and the feelings associated with it have almost equal significance. Mala (see above) could fit into this kind of profile.

Josh's condition is more like iceberg C, because his actual stammer is quite mild, but his anxiety and fear about being heard to stammer is severe.

Covert or interiorized stammering

You may have heard, or read about, overt and covert or interiorized stammering. Overt stammering is the speech of someone who has a stammer that is out in the open. As the term suggests, interiorized or covert stammering is hidden inside the speaker and often unknown to the listener. Severe stammering cannot be hidden, but mild to moderate forms of the condition can, and are concealed from the rest of the world and kept inside the speaker by use of ingenious avoidance strategies. If you are reading this book because you stammer, then avoidance behaviour will be clear to you, but for other readers, here are just a few examples of avoidance (this topic will be discussed more fully later in the book):

Sayed does all his shopping in supermarkets, thus avoiding having to ask for items in the corner shop.

If forced to answer a question in class, Marika deliberately avoids the correct answer because it contains a sound that she finds difficult, and instead gives a wrong response that she can say easily.

Michael goes to great lengths to make sure he has the correct change so that he can avoid asking for his bus-fare.

Stammerers and fluent people alike find it difficult to understand how someone like Josh can talk absolutely fluently for long periods and then start to stammer almost out of the blue, while Mala stammers frequently, but can talk fluently to her mother and best friend. This is partly because stammering is a condition that is affected by environmental issues. It seems that the person who stammers has a slightly unstable speech mechanism so that, when everything is going well, speech can be easy and fluent. However, when speakers such as Josh or Mala perceive certain situations as 'difficult', tension creeps in, the system becomes overloaded, breaks down and stammering occurs. In Mala's case, she feels comfortable with her mother and her best friend, so her speech is easy; however, when she feels that she is being judged (whether or not this is the case is irrelevant), or when someone speaks very quickly and she feels the need to respond quickly, or when someone becomes angry or authoritarian, then this puts extra pressure on her system and speech breaks down.

The causes of stammering

Researchers agree that the causes of stammering are complex and seem to consist of a combination of different factors that interact in a variety of ways in individual speakers. It is not fully understood why some people have a more vulnerable speech system than others.

Brain imaging research has been carried out comparing those who stammer with those who do not but, because stammering is not a uniform condition, research findings may not apply to all who stammer. The differences found to date include:

- the structure and way certain areas of the brain work – as yet, it is not known whether these differences are part of the cause of stammering, or a response to it;

- fractionally slower co-ordination of muscles used in speech and voice production;
- the way that people who stammer hear their own voice while talking.

Stammering can run in families, and studies in genetics indicate that it is likely that the condition can be inherited, as can the chances of early recovery. However, some people have no family history and, in that case, other factors play a greater part in development. It is known that the possible causes of stammering are a complex combination of inherited, physical, linguistic and environmental factors, and it is the combination of these factors that is unique to every person who stammers.

The stammer and the person who stammers

There is no such thing as the typical stammer, nor is there such a person as the typical stammerer. There is a wide variety of people from all backgrounds and lifestyles who have just one thing in common – they all have some kind of interruption to the easy flow of speech and, as they get older, feel anxious about their speech; these interruptions and feelings, though, differ widely both in quantity and quality. Approximately 1 per cent of the adult population stammers – from Africa to India, from Japan to the USA and, it is thought, in every country throughout the world.

Stammering is not confined to any particular educational group, personality type or ethnicity – it is a universal difficulty with many diverse characteristics. Thinking about people who stammer as one group is a bit like classifying all red-haired people together when the only thing they might have in common would be the colour of their hair!

Stammering is a condition with many different elements. Whichever element is experienced most strongly by someone who stammers, or whatever part is heard by the listener – that is the aspect of stammering that is noted. So the most common descriptions given by people who stammer are:

- 'The word gets stuck.'
- 'I just can't say it, I get completely blocked.'
- 'I run out of breath.'
- 'I get panicky waiting to respond with my name in class when they call the register.'

- 'I know that I will have a problem when I give a presentation or talk in a group.'
- 'I never use the telephone and that makes life very difficult.'

While listeners report:

- 'It's a speech difficulty.'
- 'It's something to do with anxiety or nerves.'
- 'I think he speaks too quickly.'
- 'He's not breathing correctly.'
- 'My colleague says he stammers, but I've never heard it.'

As stated, we know that stammering is not a unitary, homogeneous, identical or uniform condition. It is extremely variable – children and adults alike can be fluent for a period of an hour, a day or a week and then start to stammer again – often without knowing the reason for their speech difficulty recurring.

Main points in this chapter

- 'Stammer' and 'stutter' are two words that mean exactly the same thing.
- Stammering is not a single, identical or homogeneous condition. It covers a wide range of difficulties from severe to mild.
- The causes of stammering are complex and individual.
- There is no such thing as the typical stammer.
- There is no such person as the typical stammerer.
- The 'icebergs' of stammering are useful in explaining that a stammer consists of two aspects – the speech behaviour (overt) and the hidden feelings (covert).
- Stammering is often misunderstood – by the speaker and the listener – because it is thought to consist solely of the speech difficulty, while the hidden feelings of older children and adults are not recognized.
- It is a highly variable condition. People can be fluent for hours, days or weeks and then start to stammer again. *That* is stammering!

2

The early stages

This chapter is addressed to parents, carers, pre-school staff, childminders and all who are concerned with the speech of young children.

As was mentioned in Chapter 1, stammering is a highly individual condition, so although the information and advice we are giving in this chapter is generally applicable and accepted, not everything stated will be relevant to everyone.

Recovery from stammering

About 5 per cent of young children begin to stammer, but some only stammer for a few weeks before they become fluent. More boys stammer than girls because girls generally find learning to talk easier.

It is thought that four out of five who stammer in childhood recover naturally, although it may take up to 18 months or longer for that recovery to occur. Some children seem more likely to recover than others:

- More girls recover than boys.
- Those who have family members who recovered naturally.
- Those who learn to talk at an average age – that is, neither markedly late nor significantly early.

It can be reassuring to know that the severity of early stammering has no bearing on the likelihood of recovery – those who stammer severely can recover naturally within a few months.

Stammering or normal hesitations

While they are learning to talk, most small children produce speech that is hesitant and lacking in fluency because the process of acquiring speech is complicated. In order to produce easy, fluent speech we must be able to put our thoughts into words, put the words into grammatical sentences, and arrange the sounds in the words in the right order, co-ordinating breathing and voice with the muscles required to articulate sounds. It is not surprising that this finely balanced act of co-ordination can break down, under certain circumstances, in young children who are still acquiring the necessary skills.

Those who are having trouble learning to talk may find it particularly hard to express all their ideas and, in their effort to be understood, their fluency can suffer. Children who learn to speak earlier than usual can also be more susceptible to stammering because they try to say very difficult things while their ability to talk is still new and unstable.

As adults we hesitate, repeat words and say 'um' and 'er' when we are tired, stressed or trying to do too many things at once. It is to be expected that children, in the process of acquiring the skills of talking, will also do this.

The types of hesitancies that are quite usual in young children (and sometimes in adults) include the following:

- Saying 'um' or 'er' when deciding what to say.
- Repeating a few words together – for example, 'Can we go ... can we go to the park, Mummy?'
- Saying whole words or parts of words two or three times – for example, 'Can ... can ... can we go to the park?' or 'Ca ... ca ... can we go to the park?'

It is less common for young children to stretch out a sound in a word – for example, 'Ssssssee that boat, Daddy?' It is very rare for them to hold tightly on to a sound with too much tension in their mouths or vocal cords in the throat. These two types of speech difficulty are more likely to occur in those who are stammering.

It is not just the type of speech disruption that indicates that a child may be stammering, as compared to being normally hesitant. The number of times the disruptions occur may also suggest the early stages of stammering. We all hesitate occasionally, but someone who stammers may do so many times in a conversation. For example, Shaheed, age three, repeated words two or three times, but he did this so often that his parents became concerned:

'Mum ... Mum ... Mum I ... I can't get this to ... to ... to work. Does ... does it ... it ... it go this ... this ... this way?'

Sometimes Shaheed would repeat a word so many times that his parents became certain that this was not usual for children of his age:

'My ... my ... my ... my ... my ... my ... my ... my ... my ... my car's gone.'

Speech and language therapy (SLT)

If you are concerned about a child's fluency, early referral is advisable. Speech and language therapists (SLTs) like to see children who stammer as young as is possible, even if there is no need for any immediate help and recovery occurs naturally. Parents can usually refer their child directly to local speech and language therapy in the UK, but there may be a waiting list for assessment. The British Stammering Association (BSA) can be contacted for a list of SLTs who specialize in stammering.

The therapist will be able to advise on whether there are indications of early stammering, and whether natural recovery is likely to occur. You will be offered advice on the best type of help for your child, and this can include:

- careful monitoring until natural reduction occurs;
- establishing the situations that lead to stammering and experimenting with ways you can help;
- working on language development or speech sounds to resolve any difficulties or delay;
- demonstrating how to reinforce the times when speech is easy in order to increase fluency and decrease stammering;
- helping the child to talk more smoothly through using toys or cartoon characters as illustrations.

In pre-school children, before the stammer has become too established, the therapist may suggest using the Lidcombe Program. This was developed in Australia and is increasingly popular in both the UK and USA, but it has to be delivered by a SLT who has had special training. The Lidcombe Program trains parents to deliver therapy that systematically reinforces fluent speech, and gently discourages stammered speech, helping the child to 'fix bumpy words'.

You may be unable to see a SLT for a variety of reasons, or experience a considerable waiting period. Here are some ways to support your child in the meantime. None of these suggestions can cause harm, or aggravate the speech situation; on the contrary, whether there is early stammering or not, the strategies below will be of considerable help to all children.

Gather information

Start by listening to both the stammer and the fluency objectively. How much variation is there from situation to situation? What factors seem to affect the speech? Is speech easier when talking to some people than others?

If possible, keep a daily diary about fluency. It has proved useful to give each day a fluency rating between 0 and 10, 0 being no stammering, and 10 being the most you have ever heard the child stammer. You can take an average over the whole day and, if there are others who you would like to involve (e.g. grandparents, nursery staff or child-minders), you could discuss the day's ratings with them and consider whether they agree with your findings. You can simply note the rating out of 10 on your calendar each day, or some people like to put an X on a chart (see Appendix A) so that they can see, at a glance, how the fluency is rising or falling. We have provided a blank chart which you can use or copy (see Appendix B).

Carrying out this exercise can act as a reminder to listen each day to the child's speech and acknowledge the days that have lots of fluency, as well as the ones where there is more stammering. We often do not really hear, or remember, the fluent speech because we take it so much for granted, only focusing on the days when the stammer is more frequent. Here is one parent's experience:

> I was really worried about Charlie's stammer and was very aware when it was happening. When I took the trouble to write down each day how much he was stammering and how much he was fluent, I realized that he wasn't stammering all the time and could go for days without stammering much at all. I wasn't really aware of that before I started to keep the diary. It has also helped me to start to think about why he is stammering more on some days than others.

Factors that may affect fluency

At the same time as keeping a daily rating chart or diary, you could write down what the child was doing, and who else was present, during a fluent period, as well as when there was loss of fluency or stammering. This exercise can indicate factors that may contribute to the breakdown in the child's speech. These factors will be individual to each child, but below are some of the most common ones:

- The child is feeling tired or ill.
- The child is excited.
- There are lots of people talking at once.
- The child is talking to an adult who is looking away – for example, the adult may be driving.
- The adults and older children are talking very quickly.

- The child is being asked lots of questions.
- The child is being asked to stand up and tell a story about an event.
- The child is talking about an event that was upsetting.
- The child is describing something that is very complicated.
- There are significant changes going on – like moving house, a new baby or starting school.

Noting down any factors that you think may affect fluency can help because you can experiment with changing some of the situations that cause difficulty, and find out whether such changes enable more fluency. There will be some situations that you can change relatively easily – like not telling a child about an exciting party or holiday until near to the day. You may find this hard because part of the pleasure of such events is to enjoy the build-up together; however, you may decide that, if it helps with fluency, it is worth doing for a short period until the language and speech skills strengthen sufficiently to cope with adverse situations without loss of speech control.

Other situations are not as easy to change, such as being unable to look at the child who is speaking because you are driving the car. You may be able to find ways round this – perhaps playing a favourite song or story cassette/CD so you can sing along together rather than talking.

If you notice situations when there is more fluency, you can try to provide some of those experiences each day – even if just for a very short time. One parent described how she had managed to help her daughter increase her fluency in this way:

> I realized that Heather stammered most when the whole family were together. We are a very talkative family and her older brothers and sisters all talk at once, so Heather couldn't get a word in. When we were alone, having a chat or playing with her toys, she was almost completely fluent. I decided to make time every day for her to play with me or share a book on her own. I could only manage a few minutes some days, but she enjoyed this calm time together and I felt better knowing I had managed to give her some fluent speech each day.

When spending 'special time' like this, it is particularly important that you let children choose what to play or talk about, and you follow their lead. Listening to what is being said rather than how it is said is also helpful. Some 10–15 minutes spent like this may help to set the pattern for increased fluency for the rest of the day.

You cannot always work out why the stammer is more frequent, and sometimes there is no special reason. Alternatively, something may be happening within the child that we adults cannot see, or do anything about. For example, one father commented:

> I really couldn't work out why Liu had started to stammer more, because nothing had happened out of the ordinary. Then the speech and language therapist asked me whether he was talking any differently recently. His mother and I had both noticed that over the last few weeks he was using lots of new words and longer sentences. He seemed to be talking non-stop. The therapist thought that this sudden growth in his talking could have caused the increased stammering and that it should settle down once he had more practice at using the new words and longer sentences.

In addition to managing some of the situations that affect your child's fluency, you can use the strategies below that help to keep children calm, reassure them that you are listening, and offer gentle support.

Be a good listener

SLTs are often asked, 'What am I supposed to do when a child stammers?' Individuals differ, and you know how best to handle awkward situations – the stammer is not so different from these other times. Here are some ideas that many have found useful:

- Wait until what is being said is complete.
- Try to stay relaxed.
- If possible, get down to children's level rather than towering above them.
- Resist the urge to interrupt or complete the sentence.
- Show interest in what is being said by maintaining eye contact.

Looking and waiting will give the impression that there is no rush and that you want to hear what is being said. Every parent knows it is not always possible to stop what you are doing and listen fully to children. There are times when you have to hurry them along to get to school on time or carry out jobs that demand your full attention. You will need to decide when you can stop what you are doing for a moment to look and listen because that will help fluency, as well as reducing the times when you have to ask them to wait until you are ready.

Like everyone else, children who stammer need to learn to take turns at talking and, as they get older, we expect them to learn how to be polite, to wait for adults to finish, and not to interrupt. You still need to help a child who stammers to learn these social rules as children cannot dominate a conversation just because they stammer.

Reducing time pressure

People often talk more quickly if they are being hurried and others around them are speaking fast. Creating an atmosphere where the child feels less rushed may indirectly slow speech down and thus increase fluency. Adults can help to do this in a variety of ways:

- Become more aware of rushing and time pressure and try to allow more time for tasks.
- Talk in a slightly slower way, with more pauses – this can indirectly slow down a child's speech.
- Take a small pause before responding to a question – this can help to slow a conversation down, and reduces interruptions and talking over people.

Speaking more slowly generally gives the brain and speech muscles more time to co-ordinate everything that is needed for fluent, easy speech. Using these strategies may help indirectly to reduce the rate of speech and have a beneficial effect on fluency.

In Chapter 3 we describe how directly teaching a child to talk more slowly may help, but this work will be done by the SLT in ways that can be understood by young children. New ways of speaking need a gradual approach and careful supervision. In the meantime, there are other ways you can support your child.

Giving advice

It is natural that you should try to help your child by giving advice on ways to stop the stammering. Well-meaning friends and relatives often offer suggestions, but these are usually not based on a sound understanding of the nature of early stammering. Common advice given to children includes:

- 'Stop stammering.'
- 'Stop and start again.'
- 'Slow down.'
- 'Relax.'
- 'Take a deep breath.'
- 'Try a different word.'

On the whole, giving such advice while the child is speaking is unhelpful because it:

- interrupts the flow of speech, making the task of putting thoughts into words even harder;
- is not usually understood by very young children who do not know how to alter their rate of speech or breathe differently;
- gives the message that stammering is wrong and builds up the underneath part of the 'stammering iceberg'.

Remember that stammering is happening for a variety of different reasons and will take time to resolve.

Give reassurance

Many young children remain unaware, and unconcerned, about their early stammering. If they appear frustrated or upset about their stammering, feel free to talk about it and give them reassurance that speech can 'get a little bumpy' when learning to talk. You would offer reassurance and encouragement if there was difficulty learning to ride a bike or putting a fiddly toy together. Listen to how the child is describing the speech difficulty and use his words when you talk about it – he may describe the stammer as 'getting stuck' or 'hard words'.

Some children tell you clearly that they cannot talk properly, or ask you to say a word for them. But distress at stammering can also be shown in more subtle ways, such as giving up talking, keeping quiet, changing words, putting on a different voice or whispering. Reassurance and encouragement to go ahead and speak anyway can help to maintain a child's confidence in talking. Tell the child that you will listen to her and that you can go to see someone (the SLT) who can help people with talking, and that it will get easier.

Parents who stammer

If you stammer yourself, you will be able to be particularly understanding and supportive of your child. Do not be afraid to let your child hear you stammer. Be reassured that children do not learn stammering from others and will not copy stammering in the long term. If you can demonstrate that you feel comfortable about your stammer by looking relaxed and confident while talking, then this will help to give your child confidence to talk, regardless of whether or not stammering occurs.

Help for more established stammering

If a child has been stammering for a long time or has become aware, frustrated and upset by stammering, the strategies in this chapter will still be helpful, but the SLT may also need to give more direct help. The next chapter provides information on how this can be done.

Main points in this chapter

- Recovery from stammering.
- Normal hesitations.
- How and when to refer to a SLT.
- SLT approaches, including the Lidcombe Program.
- How to keep a daily diary.
- Managing factors that affect fluency.
- Good listening and reducing time pressure.
- Giving advice to the child is usually not helpful.
- Ways of offering reassurance.
- Parents who stammer.

3

Established stammering

In Chapter 2 we suggested ways that adults can support children who are in the early stages of stammering and who are quite likely to regain fluent speech. In this chapter we will describe how speech and language therapy (SLT) can help children whose stammer has become more established and, possibly, more complex.

Awareness of the stammer

Individual children vary as to how soon they become aware of their stammer. Some very young children may be so frustrated that they give up talking or ask their parents to talk for them, while other older children are only vaguely conscious of how they talk, and remain unconcerned. It is often assumed that, if there is awareness, then distress must also be present, but this is not necessarily true.

Talking about stammering

It is useful to know whether or not a child is aware or distressed because the level of help that is appropriate is partly dependent on this issue. If your child talks about having difficulty speaking and asks for help, then you will be given insight into the situation but, frequently, for any number of reasons, children do not discuss this subject. Here are some more subtle signs of growing awareness and/or concern. For example, on certain occasions, does your child:

- talk in a different voice or whisper;
- pretend not to know a word or change a word;
- keep quiet or try to avoid talking;
- tap or hit something to help the word come out?

These are some of the tricks or strategies that children may use in order to reduce the stammer because they:

- do not like the physical feeling of words getting stuck;
- are frustrated at not being able to get their message across;

- are becoming aware that other people react negatively when they stammer.

Changes in the type of stammering can also indicate that the child is attempting different ways to help the words come out more easily. When a word feels stuck in the mouth or throat, it is natural to try to push it out more forcefully and hurry it along. Unfortunately, both rushing and pushing the speech muscles tightly together make it more difficult to co-ordinate the movements necessary for smooth, easy speech. These strategies are not helpful in the long term because they make the difficulty more complex.

Speech and language therapy (SLT)

As stammering becomes more established, negative thoughts and feelings tend to develop. A child may feel helpless, frustrated and different to others, and the bottom of the 'iceberg' described in Chapter 1 begins to form. Timely intervention by a SLT can provide more helpful ways of managing the stammer, as well as preventing the development of some unnecessary aspects.

SLTs have access to various therapy programmes which, according to the age and interests of the child, may use stories, toys or cartoon characters to illustrate the techniques being taught.

In the case of older children, their views are crucial as to when and how therapy is delivered. Some children ask clearly for help, others are really not concerned about their stammer and do not find it to be a problem. In this case, the SLT may recommend postponing therapy until they are ready, as unwanted therapy can be counterproductive.

The aims of therapy

For older children whose stammers are more complicated and of longer standing, the final outcome of therapy varies. Some will eventually recover and become completely fluent. A small percentage will continue to stammer and, in therapy, will be helped to manage their speech. In general, therapy aims to help children to:

- feel good about talking, stammering and themselves;
- be able to understand their stammer and know that, on occasions, even fluent speakers hesitate and stumble;
- use techniques to increase fluency, as well as to stammer in a relaxed, easy way;
- become confident and effective communicators.

Most programmes followed by a SLT share elements that are described below. Which elements are used and in which order will depend upon the individual needs and preferences of the child, the parents and others who are involved.

New speaking skills need to be established very slowly with lots of daily practice, in fun activities, using gradually longer sentences and when talking to different people. Once the skills become easy and effortless, the SLT will advise on how to transfer these speaking techniques to everyday situations.

Fluency is not the only goal of therapy. Natural fluency is unattainable for some children, however hard they try and however much help they receive from parents and a therapist. These children need to be equipped to deal effectively with their speech, and to feel good about themselves so that they can succeed in life regardless of their stammers.

Understanding speaking and stammering

Many therapy programmes start with a simple explanation of how both breathing and the speech muscles are used to produce speech. Most children have only a vague awareness of how they stammer and it is helpful to let them explore their stammers and become more aware of what they do in their individual stammering patterns. This is done in a gently supportive way; for example, the child can 'catch' pretend stammers in a SLT's speech, listen to recordings of speech, and finally catch and describe various types of stammering that occur while talking.

This type of work, which increases awareness and understanding of what people do when they stammer, has two positive effects. As the stammer is explored with an emotionally calm yet interested therapist, the mysteries of the stammer are explained and the child starts to feel less helpless and more in control of his speech. As the unnecessary tricks are exposed, it becomes evident that these may not be useful, and the child is ready to try different ways of changing speech that are more effective.

It is also usual to encourage children to listen to the speech of fluent people to discover that everyone stumbles over words and hesitates sometimes. This work ensures that children who stammer have realistic goals and are comfortable with the normal 'ums', 'ers' and hesitations in their speech.

Once children know what they do when, and because they stammer, they are ready to try out new ways of speaking. These are often referred to as fluency techniques or speech modification techniques.

Speech modification techniques

These fall into two categories:

1 Ways to increase fluency.
2 Ways to ease through stammers smoothly.

Both techniques aim to counteract the tension and rushing that have built up as unhelpful coping strategies, and they usually involve slower and more relaxed ways of speaking that can be shaped towards natural-sounding speech.

Increasing overall fluency generally involves teaching the child to speak more slowly, flow words together, and make sounds loosely in the mouth and throat. If easing through tense stammers is the approach chosen, children will practise catching the stammer and then moving through it easily and gently.

Which of the above approaches is selected for the child depends on the type of stammer. Many older children are taught both techniques so that they are enabled to increase their fluency, and also have a 'safety-net' technique to deal with any stammers that occur. The skills involved are very similar, and many children quickly become adept at using both approaches in order to talk more fluently and ease through any remaining stammers.

Maria, eight, describes how she manages her speech:

It's easier now because I can talk more slowly and I know how to use a slide if I get stuck. If I'm with my friends, I don't mind if I stammer and I just talk. But if I'm answering a question in class or I feel a bit nervous, I can slow down and slide my stammers. I know how to help my stammer if I need to – so I join in more now.

Reducing avoidance

As children become more confident in using their new techniques to make speaking easier, they will be encouraged to try some of the words and speaking situations that they have avoided due to a fear of stammering. They will be helped to approach these in a systematic way, starting with the easiest, least frightening situations.

Some of these speaking situations will be at school and the teacher can play an important role by supporting the child and working with the SLT so that full participation in classroom and whole-school activities can ultimately be achieved.

General communication skills

Being fluent is not necessary for good communication. There are people who stammer who are easy to listen to and who are good at getting their message across, and there are fluent people who are boring and poor communicators. It is important to help children to understand that good communication depends on more than fluency, and to provide them with skills that will turn them into people who can communicate well – regardless of whether or not they stammer.

Therapy often includes information and practice on social skills such as:

- Posture
- Observation
- Eye contact
- Listening skills
- Taking turns
- How to start conversations
- Problem solving
- Negotiation skills
- Giving talks.

Children who stammer may have missed out on opportunities to develop these abilities. Given the chance to develop in this area, they have the potential to become better communicators than some of their fluent peers, which will give them an advantage in education, and later in the workplace.

Building self-confidence

In Chapter 11 we describe how thoughts and self-talk affect feelings and, eventually, self-confidence. Many of the strategies described can be adapted by SLTs in their work with children to prevent the vicious cycle of anxiety and worsening stammering.

One of the simplest ways that parents and teachers can improve children's self-talk and increase their self-esteem is to use praise effectively.

Praise is most effective when it is specific and describes what the child has done well. For example, saying a vague 'Good girl' or 'Well done' does not tell the child exactly what she has done well. It is better to be more specific and build up a vocabulary of characteristics that the child can apply to herself, such as 'I am helpful/kind/brave/a good swimmer'.

You can do this by wording praise in the following ways:

- Describe what the child has done: 'Well done, James, you have put all your things away in the cupboard' or 'Thank you for helping Tom when he fell over in the playground'.
- Now add a word that describes the action and that can be applied to the child: 'That was very organized of you' or 'You are very kind'.

Those with low self-confidence can find it hard to think of positive things that they have done and been praised for. Children can make a 'Praise Scrapbook' where they write down nice things that people have said about them, and then draw a picture to go with it. Alternatively, they can write achievements on pieces of paper to keep in a special 'Praise Box'.

Group therapy

Attending SLT with a group of children of a similar age can be very powerful because joining with others, who have similar difficulties, is supportive and reduces feelings of being different and 'the only one'. A group may provide the first opportunity to meet others who stammer, and a greater range of therapy activities can be provided than on a one-to-one basis – making the experience more fun.

Group therapy is held on a weekly basis or intensively where the children attend every day for a week or more during the school holidays. Therapists in the UK can also refer children to specialist SLT centres that offer intensive therapy further away from home. Some of these courses are residential and incorporate outdoor adventure activities to build self-confidence and group skills. Other centres offer support to the families of those who stammer and run a parents' group alongside the group for children. More information about specialist centres in the UK is available from the BSA, or by looking on their website for links.

There are also some non-SLT group therapy courses that are advertised. These courses are run by non-professionals – often it is people who stammered themselves and now run groups to help others. These approaches were originally designed for adults and some have found them to be very helpful. We would advocate caution about enrolling children and teenagers on to such courses without ensuring that they are suitable for your child's age group and stammering pattern.

Teachers

It can be very helpful for the teacher and therapist to work closely together to support the child who stammers. When at all possible, the SLT will consult school staff during assessment and liaise regularly during therapy.

Teachers usually have a number of children with additional educational needs in their classrooms and are skilled at modifying classroom routines to accommodate differences in children. Situations that can prove challenging for pupils who stammer include registration, reading aloud, drama and speaking in class or larger gatherings, such as assembly.

Professionals can feel unsure about whether they should talk openly about the stammer for fear of causing embarrassment. Teachers should be reassured that it is best to talk to the child directly about their stammer – but to do so in private. Reassurance can be offered that they are aware of the stammer and will help when needed. The type of help will depend entirely upon the child. Some children wish to be included in all activities regardless of their stammer, while others prefer not to be asked to read aloud or talk in front of the whole class.

Here is one teacher's experience:

> At first Aiden was reluctant to speak at all in front of the group so we had a talk and came up with some alternative ways of doing things. I changed registration for all the children to just putting up a hand when I called their name – this helped Aiden and also a couple of other children who have communication difficulties. Aiden is happier talking in unison with other people, so he reads aloud with another child and we also used paired speaking for assemblies. Aiden enjoys drama, but chose non-speaking or singing parts initially. As Aiden's stammer improved, I checked whether he wanted to try to do some things by himself and he has now started talking and answering questions in a small group. His confidence is improving gradually, but it is a slow process.

Although individual children have different needs, below are some general tips for teachers that will help all children who stammer:

- Keep eye contact even if the child looks away while stammering.
- Give time to finish without interrupting or hurrying the child along.
- If possible, speak in an unhurried way.
- Do not give advice such as 'slow down' or 'relax'.

- Have a one-to-one conversation about how to help in the classroom.

There are specific leaflets, books and websites that give information addressed to teachers, and some are listed in Further reading and Useful addresses at the back of this book. The BSA has sent a CD-Rom to all schools in the UK, providing information and guidelines for supporting those who stammer in the classroom and during oral examinations.

Teasing and bullying

Alec, age nine, described how he was teased at school:

> He would say words over and over and over in a silly voice and call me 'stutter boy'. Once he was doing it in the dinner line and I couldn't get away. I got so mad that I hit him hard and the teacher saw me and I got into trouble. I was so angry I couldn't talk to her, and just went off by myself into a corner of the playground.

Teasing or bullying can be verbal, physical or emotional. It can happen to children who are younger, smaller, or have something different about them, like wearing glasses or coming first in various subjects. It is possible that a child will be teased about his stammer, although this is not inevitable. There are many publications and websites that offer sound advice to children, parents and teachers about how to handle bullying (see Further reading and Useful addresses).

Here are some general guidelines for adults about managing teasing and bullying:

- If you suspect, ask directly.
- Find out about the school's anti-bullying policy. All state schools must, by law, have this policy.
- Discuss possible ways of dealing with the situation, but allow the child to make the final choice about which of these to implement.

Here are some suggestions for children:

- Don't react. Bullying is no fun for the bully if the child does not cry or fight back. Try to react as if the bullying is childish and make any responses in a calm voice.
- Don't argue, just agree. The lack of argument will make the bully bored and give up. Say calmly 'I know I stammer and that's OK' or 'If you say so' or 'Yes, I stammer'.

- Use a sense of humour and make a clever remark: 'I'm trying to win the prize for the longest sentence'.
- Practise what you are going to say in the mirror, with your parents and friends. Try standing tall and firm, as well as responding with a calm voice.
- Tell a parent, teacher, friendly adult, older friend or sibling. They should not take over, but ask you what you want to happen.
- Keep a journal. Write down when, where, who did what, who else saw, and who was told. This can build up evidence to show how serious and constant bullying can be.

Main points in this chapter

- The aims of speech and language therapy (SLT).
- Therapy techniques.
- Using praise to build self-confidence.
- Group therapy can be powerful.
- How teachers can help.
- Dealing with teasing.

4

Teenagers and young adults

This chapter is about young people who are in the transition period of their lives between childhood and adulthood. The text is addressed to the young person who stammers, but will also be of help to parents and teachers of this age group.

A time of change

This period of life involves many changes – in body size and shape, hormonal activity that can affect emotions and moods, and the development of new interests and social circles. Teenagers gradually become increasingly independent of their parents.

You may be reading this chapter as a young teenager who is trying to do more things by yourself, or as an older teenager or young adult who is already living alone without much support from family members. Some young people fall out with their parents over how much they can do by themselves, while others turn to their parents for help and advice. Everyone is different.

As you become more independent of your parents, your friends have probably become increasingly important and sexual relationships create new challenges. Secondary school education brings pressure to do well in exams, and options over subjects that affect future job prospects. Decisions arise as to what sort of career to choose.

Facing these new situations can be challenging enough without having to deal with your speech. In this chapter we will discuss ways you can help yourself manage your stammering so that it does not get in the way of decisions you are making about your future. We will also tell you which parts of this book can help you with your stammer at the present time.

You may have had SLT at a younger age and this might have been useful, but you now need some extra ideas to help you with new situations that you are facing in education or the workplace. Children are often told that they will grow out of stammering and you could now be wondering why it has not disappeared, and what you can do about it. Strategies learned at an earlier stage may not now be sufficient, and you could be looking for something different. It may help you to think about what you want from this book by writing in the box below why you are reading it, and what you hope to gain.

What I hope to gain

If you have read the book from the start, you will have discovered that most young children recover from stammering, but that the older you are the less likely it is that you will recover completely. Your stammer might be here to stay, and that could be a disappointing or frightening prospect for you. The good news is that there is much you can do to help yourself, and that many adults live successfully with their stammers and do the jobs they want as teachers, policemen and policewomen, actors, plumbers – in fact, people who stammer can be found in almost every field of employment.

Many of the following chapters on how adults can help themselves to manage their stammering will be relevant to you. For now, we will stay with issues that are specific to you as a young person.

Secondary school

The move from primary or junior school to secondary school can be a daunting one. You are moving from a small, safe community where you know most of the children, and the teachers know you. Once you arrive at secondary school you will probably find that it's much larger and has many children you have not met before. Rather than being taught by one teacher who knows you well, you will be taught by many different teachers. It is harder for them to get to know you, and it can be difficult to tell them about your stammer and how they can help you with it in school.

One of the ways you might be coping with your stammer may be to hide it, but certain ways of hiding a stammer can cause other problems. Here are some young people's experiences:

> Suzanne, age 13: 'I am so afraid of stammering in class that I keep as quiet as I can. I never volunteer to answer a question, which really bugs me as I often know the answer. If one of the teachers picks on me and I think I'll stammer, I sometimes give a wrong answer that I can say without stammering. I hate it that the other people think I am stupid – but it's better than them seeing me stammer because then I go all red and feel really embarrassed.'

Ross, age 15: 'If I am going to be forced to take a turn to speak, I will do something that I know will get me thrown out of class. I'll throw something at someone else or pick a fight. I get lots of detentions and my parents get really angry with me. I sometimes feel really down that they don't know the real reason why I do these things.'

Jamal, age 17: 'I had a lot of bullying because of my stammer when I was younger and I've learnt how to play the class joker. If I make the class laugh by swearing or being rude it distracts everyone from my stammer, but it can get me into trouble. Sometimes I feel like I never get the chance to be the real me.'

There are some ways that may make it easier to tell the teachers the things they need to know about your stammer. Your parents could help you with this, or you might want to do it alone. If your parents, or your therapist, do talk to the teachers, then it is important that you go to the meetings too so that you can begin to take responsibility for decisions that are made. It also shows the teachers that the first person they should ask about your stammer is you – you know most about it. Here are some suggestions as to how you can tell teachers about your stammer and about the help they can give you:

- Try to find out if there is one teacher whose job it is to tell all the others about any children who have special educational needs. You may require special consideration in class and during some exams that involve speaking. This teacher would be a good one to go to first and will know the best way of passing on your wishes to all the other teachers.
- If there is no such teacher in your school, or you find it too difficult to talk to this person, you may want to talk to a teacher who you particularly like or who already knows about your stammer, and ask them to tell the other teachers.
- If you find talking too difficult, you could write down what you think the teacher needs to know. For example, you could use the headings in the box below.

Some subjects have oral exams which involve speaking in a foreign language with your teacher, or giving a presentation to the class. This could be hard for you, or you may even avoid taking that subject altogether because you cannot face an oral exam. You are allowed to ask that the exam be carried out in a slightly different way than that for the other pupils, to make sure that you can show the examiners what you know and be marked like all the other students.

Things my teacher needs to know

To my teacher (teacher's name)
From (your name)

Please give this to all the teachers who teach me.

I have written down some things about my stammer that I hope will be useful. I would like to talk to you about my stammer once you have had a chance to read this.

I do this when I stammer:

I find it hard to talk in the following situations:

I do these things so people won't notice that I am stammering:

When I am speaking I would like you to:

It is not helpful when I am speaking if you:

If you see others laugh, tease or bully me about my stammer, I would like you to:

I have found the following books and websites about stammering useful:

If you are not sure how to help me, please ask me. I would prefer to do this in private rather than in front of the class. Thank you.

One pupil, Alberto, described how his school handled an oral exam differently:

> I was terrified of giving a presentation to the whole class as part of the English exam. My therapist came with me to meet my teacher and we talked about how to handle the oral exam. I

explained that I would stammer very badly if I had to do it in front of the whole class. My teacher asked how many people I would be comfortable talking to and we decided that I should give the presentation to the teacher and four of my close friends who I don't stammer very much with. I felt quite happy with this and felt that I could give as good a talk as the other students by doing it in this way. The teacher also asked my therapist to write a letter for the exam board explaining why I needed special consideration for my stammer.

Bullying

If you are having trouble with other children laughing at your stammer or bullying, you will find helpful information in: Chapter 3, Further reading and also Useful addresses.

Starting college, university or work

When applying for a job or a place at university you will face selection procedures such as application forms and possibly interviews. You may be anxious that your stammer will be a disadvantage or could even prevent you from being successful. You can include the fact that you stammer in your application form or mention it to the university admissions officer. Employers and universities are expected to find out from all applicants if they require special consideration or support both during the selection process and while studying or working.

Liu describes how he handled his first job application:

I was nervous about admitting that I had a stammer when I was completing the application form for a job. I described how I stammered more when I was nervous and under pressure and was therefore likely to stammer severely during the interview. Someone from the human resources department contacted me before the interview to ask if there was anything they could do to help. We agreed on extra time for the interview and this helped me to feel less pressurized on the day. In the event I performed well, despite stammering a lot at the beginning, and I was offered the job. It was also helpful because my manager knew that I stammered, and because we had discussed it openly from the start, I always felt able to talk to her if I had difficulties.

Similarly, universities will want to do all they can to assist you in doing your best academically. It is helpful to discuss your stammer with your personal tutor or course tutor so that there is some understanding of stammering, and of how it may impact on oral exams and presentations. Each university has a Student Services Department whose role it is to support all students, including those with a disability. They will be happy to talk with you and with your tutors, if necessary, about ways to give you an equal chance to show your abilities. This may include adjusting course assessments, giving more time in oral exams, or suggesting alternative ways of making presentations.

Should you face any difficulties or discrimination because of your stammer, the UK Disability Discrimination Act (1995) can sometimes cover stammering. Further information and a useful website can be found at the end of Chapter 12.

Of course, doing well academically is only one of the challenges faced by students starting at university or college. You will also be making new friends and perhaps living independently for the first time. It is comforting to know that everyone else is looking for friendship too and the first weeks of term provide many activities designed to help you to meet other students. You will find that universities are not like school, and that young adults are generally more accepting of differences in other people.

Magda, 18, described her experiences:

> I found that people didn't care that I stammered. They were only interested in me as a person and whether I was good to hang out with. A few people even asked me openly about my stammer as we were getting to know each other which made the whole thing more relaxed.

Feeling isolated

Stammering can sometimes be hard to talk about with friends. Although there are probably other young people at your school or college who stammer, it is common never to have met another young person with this sort of speech. Therefore, you can feel isolated as far as your stammer is concerned. It can be tough for your friends to appreciate how you feel about talking on the phone, answering in class, asking for a bus-fare and talking to a boy or girl you want to ask out on a date. If you ever get the chance to meet up with others who stammer, you will find it really helpful.

Associations for those who stammer usually support self-help groups, and hold email lists and telephone groups for adults and young people who stammer. Some have specific pages on their websites for teenagers and young people and you may be able to email or phone others of your age, even if you cannot meet them in person. Social networking sites can also be useful in communicating and exchanging information with other young adults who stammer.

In some areas, SLTs offer group therapy for teenagers and there are specialist centres in the UK that run intensive group therapy for up to two weeks in length. Some combine therapy with other confidence-building experiences such as outdoor adventure activities. You can locate these courses via the BSA website.

Another way of reducing your feelings of isolation can be to try and tell others more about yourself. You may be reluctant to do this because you feel that they will not be interested, or that you are making too much of your stammer. The only way to find out what their reaction is going to be is to try it out on a friendly person first. Often people are interested in stammering, but have never asked you about it because they do not want to embarrass you. If you start to talk about your stammer more and show them you want to explain it to them, you may be pleasantly surprised. Some people will even want to look at this book, or you could show them certain parts to help them understand specific aspects – like the 'stammering iceberg'.

How much you tell others or ask for their support is up to you. You can try things out for yourself or it can be helpful to work through some of the chapters in this book with the support of others.

Being a good communicator

As well as working directly on the stammer, it is a good idea to improve your general social skills. There is more to talking than just fluency. Think about who you enjoy talking to. Do you like talking with them because they:

- have interesting things to say;
- have a laugh;
- are interested when you have something to say;
- can talk things through when you disagree or need to solve a problem together?

Think of people you don't like talking to. Do they:

- talk endlessly about themselves without checking you are interested;
- hardly say anything and sit in silence;

- seem uninvolved in what you are telling them;
- refuse to talk or shout at you if there is a problem?

You will have noticed that stammering doesn't appear on either list. Just because people speak fluently does not automatically make them good communicators and, just because you stammer, this does not automatically mean that you are a bad communicator. Think about yourself as a communicator – that is, someone who gets his or her message across effectively. If you put your stammer on one side, which of the points on the above lists would you tick as being applicable to yourself?

Good general communication skills can help you to cope with new situations, succeed in the workplace and make new friends. You may not have had many opportunities to develop these skills because of your stammer, but improving in this area could increase your confidence generally.

In Further reading there are suggested books that can help you to become a better communicator by using body language, improving listening skills, having more successful conversations, and behaving assertively when there is a problem. You may want to read some of them as well as the chapters in this book about self-help.

Changing your speech

If you want to change the way you speak and to cope better with your stammer, you will find the following chapters (primarily written for adults) appropriate. They will help you understand more about your stammer, and about the things you do because you stammer. You can then decide how you want to change, and begin work on some of the ways of speaking more fluently or with easier stammers.

Main points in this chapter

- A changing time of life.
- Coping with secondary school, university and starting work.
- The Disability Discrimination Act.
- Feelings of isolation and help from others.
- Good communication skills.
- Useful chapters to help you work on stammering.

5

An introduction to therapy for adults

Therapy for stammering can be likened to the experience of rowing across an unknown lake. When you start rowing, you are fresh and enthusiastic and you row away with happy determination. Then you get halfway across the lake and you cannot see the shore from where you came and cannot see the shore to which you are heading. This can be a worrying time – 'Should I have embarked on this journey?', 'Where am I going?', 'Am I going in the right direction?', 'Have I got enough strength left?', 'I might have been better off staying where I was!' Many questions and doubts can go through your mind. This is the time to stay positive and row as hard as is possible because, very soon, the other shore will come into view and you will know where you are going. When you get to the other shore, all the rowing, the hard work, the successes and the failures of the journey will have been worthwhile.

Stammering therapy is somewhat like rowing across that unknown lake!

Starting therapy

Therapists are often asked about the exact nature of their programme, whether the stammer will be cured, and how long the therapy will take. It is virtually impossible to give precise answers to such questions because therapy evolves, and does not consist of a fixed set of stages that are followed, regardless of the needs of individual clients. The most effective therapy has clear goals, but does not follow a rigid, pre-set programme because clients have different needs and their reactions to therapy differ. Some would like more fluency, while others want to reduce the amount of avoidance that they use; some want to move slowly, others want to take everything in a rush – people are individuals, and a one-size-fits-all approach is not appropriate.

For a number of adults, undertaking a course of therapy may be a new experience, while for others it is part of a long search for a solution to their difficulties. Clients may question whether it is a good idea to embark on this journey, in case things 'get worse'. They know their feelings and attitudes at the start of therapy, but they cannot project themselves forward and know how those feelings and attitudes will have changed during, and after, a course of therapy. It is well known that the actual experience of treatment will, in itself, change certain long-held beliefs and habitual behaviours – regardless of whether that treatment is for weight loss, fear of flying, giving up smoking, or dealing with a stammer.

Michael

Michael was 32 when he came to the clinic. When asked the question 'Why have you come for therapy now?', his reply was 'I had therapy when I was at school and it didn't work so I thought there was no point in coming, but perhaps things are different now so I want to give it a try. I am scared because I can get by in my job with lots of avoiding and changing words and I don't want therapy to make me worse.'

If you are in Michael's position, the crucial question is, 'What do you mean by getting worse?' People who come to therapy with those words are really presuming that their life is pretty good at the moment and, therefore, it might be better to stay exactly where they are. In reality, it is usually found that they are finding life is getting progressively more difficult and complicated – frequently because they can no longer hide their stammer and, occasionally, because the stammer is getting more severe.

After a discussion about his anxiety, Michael took the plunge and joined a one-session-per-week evening group. Three months later he wrote the following:

I almost didn't come for therapy. I hesitated for months, but finally decided to see what it was like because I had had a particularly difficult day with a customer and was tired of trying to stay fluent. If there was any help available for somebody of my age, I was going to give it a go. I have come to the class every week quite regularly and only missed one session and it has made loads of difference. I've met other people in the same state as myself and I've learnt to deal with my panic about someone hearing me stammer. I'm not fluent by any means, but I've stopped feeling so bad about my speaking and, because I have learnt a lot about it, I can now calm down and cope with lots of occasions when I would have stammered before. I still avoid some words and situations, but much less than I did before. Somehow my life has become easier.

Why do adults come for therapy?

Adults come to therapy for all sorts of reasons. In our experience the main factors are:

- Greater fluency is thought necessary for better job prospects.
- Therapy was offered in earlier years and now a 'booster' dose is needed.
- A specific occasion requires improved speech, e.g. a family celebration speech or a presentation.
- Fear of discovery by a manager or partner after constant avoidance strategies have made everyone believe that the client is a fluent speaker.
- The stammer has got worse.

Reasons for seeking help

Perhaps none of the above applies to you and you might like to write down your own reasons for seeking help because those reasons could have a bearing on the type of therapy that would be helpful:

Fluent speakers tend to believe that the aim of all stammerers is to be fluent. This is not necessarily true. When asking clients what their main target is, the most usual answers are:

- I want to be fluent.

OR

- I want to say what I want to say when I want to say it, regardless of fluency.

OR

- I want to feel less anxious about speaking even if there is the occasional stammer.

Which of these applies to you? Any of the above, or something else?

Some issues in therapy for adults

1   General

We have discussed issues that frequently require attention when working with children or teenagers, and now issues concerning adults need consideration. Adults have concerns about their jobs, relationships, financial situation, health and so forth. People who stammer are no different from those who are fluent in that, for some, every slight setback or problem impacts on their self-confidence and then on their speech, while for others quite serious difficulties can be handled and speech is hardly affected. These differences in temperament, attitude, confidence and personality are universal, but they are relevant when understanding whether or not your stammer is closely linked to stresses in life.

The descriptions of current therapy methods (Chapter 9) may sound rather cold, complicated and clinical when written down in black and white. Words cannot do justice to the therapeutic process, nor can they describe the hard work, sense of achievement and fun that can occur as you progress through therapy and feel that you are gaining control over a difficulty that you have had for many years.

2   Psychological – flight or fight

Centuries ago when our primitive ancestors were threatened by something, perhaps a dangerous animal, they were saved by an in-built survival instinct that is known as the 'flight or fight' mechanism. When we feel in great danger, what happens is that the brain triggers a release of chemicals and hormones into the body, the main one being adrenaline, and these substances give us the extra mental and physical strength to either 'run the three-minute mile' or to turn and fight. In this way we can cope with what could be a life-threatening situation.

However, when anxious, we give the wrong signals to the brain; we signal danger, and the brain interprets this as real danger and begins to release far too much adrenaline for the current situation. Breathing can become quicker and more shallow, and feelings of dizziness, sweating and general panic can occur. The brain may assess that there is a need for more oxygen so that blood pressure goes up and the heart starts to beat faster. Now your body is ready to run the 'three-minute mile' or to stand and fight a terrifying enemy. This is not going to happen. What you predict is about to happen is that some unpleasant stammering experience will occur!

The fear of stammering can be so great that the brain interprets it as a life-threatening situation and makes the correct response to an incorrect message. The unpleasant physical sensations experienced are real enough because the brain is telling your body to get ready for a great danger.

In order to cope with anxiety and panic, we need to learn to recognize the difference between real danger and perceived danger, then the brain will receive appropriate signals, and send out correct messages to our bodies.

3 Habit

Over the years people who stammer can acquire an imaginary 'filing cabinet' in their minds with 'files' marked 'Difficult', 'Threatening', 'Can't talk to', 'Always stammer with', and so on. Certain people, such as your boss, teacher or Auntie Barbara, and specific situations, such as presentations, reading aloud or making phone calls, are stored in these imaginary 'files' because it is thought that they fall into one or other of these categories. Apart from people, certain words are considered to be in the 'Difficult file' because they are overloaded with an emotional content, or with the thought that they must be spoken fluently. As these 'files' build up with experiences of stammering, the habit factor begins to creep in – 'I always stammer with ...' or 'I always stammer when ...', as in the case of the following client:

Jean

Jean taught IT, and one of the words she felt she could not say was 'mouse'. Unless we are seriously involved with IT or keep pet mice, 'mouse' is not a word that would be of great significance to most of us. It was a very important word for Jean and she would stand in a class of teenagers and say things like, 'This gadget that I am holding', or 'When we want to move the cursor, we use this item'. Jean persuaded herself that she could not say 'mouse'. She had a stammer but, by means of using considerable avoidance tactics, she never blocked in the classroom. Therefore, she was sure the pupils would think her stupid if she suddenly stammered. By avoiding the word 'mouse' time and time again, that word began to assume terrifying proportions. Before the class even started, she would worry – so it was no wonder that, when she actually came to the word 'mouse', her brain sent down anxiety signals, her vocal cords tensed and closed and ... she blocked!

Recognizing yourself

Do you recognize yourself in this section on habit?

Do you have a 'filing cabinet' in your mind?

If so, does it have a lot of files or just a few?

What labels have you given to your files?

Do your files contain words, names of people, situations or a combination of these?

What is needed in order to benefit from therapy?

A desire for change

Change is an essential part of any therapeutic process because, if you continue to do exactly what you are doing now, the result will be exactly what it is now. The desire has to come from you. Sometimes people read a self-help book, or come to therapy, because their families, line managers or partners suggest that this is what they should do. A desire for change has to come from *you*!

The ability to take risks, and the courage to try something new

Perhaps you do all your shopping in supermarkets and avoid asking for an item in a shop, or send an email rather than use the telephone. It requires courage to take a risk and try something new, perhaps to go into that shop or pick up the phone?

The capacity to deal with setbacks

The road will not always be straight and smooth. There will still be 'bad' days, but coping with those and continuing with the work will increase confidence and the ability to deal with your stammer.

Hard work and practice

At the time of writing this book, we know of no magic pills. There are no quick fixes that will give long-term relief from stammering. Hard work is always involved.

Consistent work – going step-by-step

Taking giant leaps can leave most of us flat on our faces!

Patience

Most adults will have been stammering for 15, 20 or more years – the resultant, long-term difficulty cannot be undone in 15 or 20 minutes. Change takes time.

It is useful to consider other known factors that can help or hinder success in therapy:

People who continued to stammer spent their energies on:

- Various kinds of avoidance
- Denying that they had a problem
- Looking for quick, easy cures – for example, medication, hypnosis, speech drills, etc.

People who conquered their stammering worked with issues such as:

- Talking more
- Going ahead in spite of the stammer
- Slowing down
- Keeping calm – the stammer is not the end of the world
- Not letting their stammers stop them from participating in activities
- Acknowledging that they had a stammer
- Sharing their problem (if only with one other person).

The *good* news is: you will improve, but it may take time.

Main points in this chapter

- Therapy is a process – a journey.
- The experience of therapy will change both speech patterns and attitudes.
- Issues to consider.
- Personal requirements – emotional and practical – for success in therapy.
- Aspects that can help or hinder recovery.

6

Your own 'iceberg'

This chapter is for anyone who is about to start therapy, is presently involved in a course of therapy, or has decided to work alone. Knowing your own 'iceberg' is of considerable importance because, before you can change a behaviour, you need a clear understanding of that behaviour. This rule applies to most behaviours whether that be a fear of flying, eating too many take-aways, or stammering.

In Chapter 1 we discussed the 'icebergs' of Josh and Mala. For a reminder, see Figure 6.1.

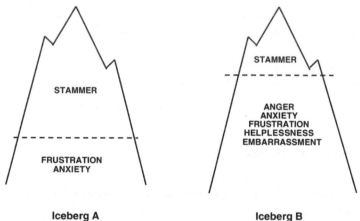

Iceberg A

Iceberg B

Mala has a severe, frequent stammer. She has learnt to live with it and so has moderate feelings of frustration and anxiety.

Josh has a mild, infrequent stammer with considerable anxiety, frustration, anger and embarrassment.

Figure 6.1   Examples of stammering 'icebergs'

The core speech behaviours are the basic and individual speech patterns that form your stammer.

Below are some questions relating to these core speech behaviours that should help you to describe the top part of the 'iceberg'. It is your own perception of your speech that is significant, so please use your own thoughts and not those of a therapist, friend or relative. Stammering is a variable condition and you may feel that your answers are dependent on the listener and the situation. If that applies to you, it would be best to choose an average.

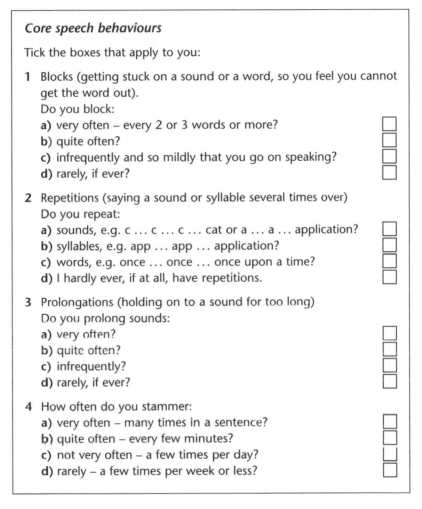

Core speech behaviours

Tick the boxes that apply to you:

1 Blocks (getting stuck on a sound or a word, so you feel you cannot get the word out).
   Do you block:
   a) very often – every 2 or 3 words or more? ☐
   b) quite often? ☐
   c) infrequently and so mildly that you go on speaking? ☐
   d) rarely, if ever? ☐

2 Repetitions (saying a sound or syllable several times over)
   Do you repeat:
   a) sounds, e.g. c ... c ... c ... cat or a ... a ... application? ☐
   b) syllables, e.g. app ... app ... application? ☐
   c) words, e.g. once ... once ... once upon a time? ☐
   d) I hardly ever, if at all, have repetitions. ☐

3 Prolongations (holding on to a sound for too long)
   Do you prolong sounds:
   a) very often? ☐
   b) quite often? ☐
   c) infrequently? ☐
   d) rarely, if ever? ☐

4 How often do you stammer:
   a) very often – many times in a sentence? ☐
   b) quite often – every few minutes? ☐
   c) not very often – a few times per day? ☐
   d) rarely – a few times per week or less? ☐

Please note that the guidelines below are just that – only guidelines. Not every profile will match our criteria. If you do not fit the general ideas outlined below, keep remembering that stammering is highly individual, and please continue to work out your own special profile.

How severe are your core stammering behaviours?

1 Blocks can be more serious than repetitions because speech is then completely stopped, and so the speaker cannot finish what is being said for the duration of that block.
2 Repetitions tend to be less serious than blocks because the speaker can continue with what is being said.
3 Prolongations vary because whether they are serious or mild depends on the amount of tension and the length of the prolongation.
4 How often you stammer is difficult to classify because, on the surface, it would seem that the more frequent the stammer, the more severe the condition. That is one circumstance, but it can be found that someone has frequent mild hesitations which are less troublesome than another person's block that is severe, but does not occur very often.

If your answers are mainly:

- (a); this indicates that at times you may have considerable difficulty when speaking because your stammer is frequent and perhaps quite severe;
- (b); this could mean that speech is affected in a moderate to severe way;
- (c); this tends to indicate a mild, infrequent stammer;
- (d); this suggests that the actual overt speech problem is relatively mild.

Now that you have thought about what you *do* (the core behaviours), it is important to examine how you *feel*.

Why is that important? You may be quite clear about the answer to this question because you have found that your stammer is influenced by the way that you feel. Alternatively, you may think that, if only you spoke fluently, your anxiety and negative feelings would just disappear. Whichever scenario you favour, it is best to understand the covert part of the 'iceberg' (the feelings) in order to have a clearer understanding of the whole stammer – rather than solely of the speech aspect. Now answer the questions on page 43.

You may have found that most of your answers are (a) or (b), in which case you seem to have quite strong feelings when you stammer, and about your stammer, whereas for mainly (c) your feelings are fairly mild, and for mainly (d) your feelings do not seem to be an important aspect of your stammering behaviour.

Does your iceberg show that you are primarily concerned about your speech (the top of the iceberg)? Or primarily concerned with your nega-

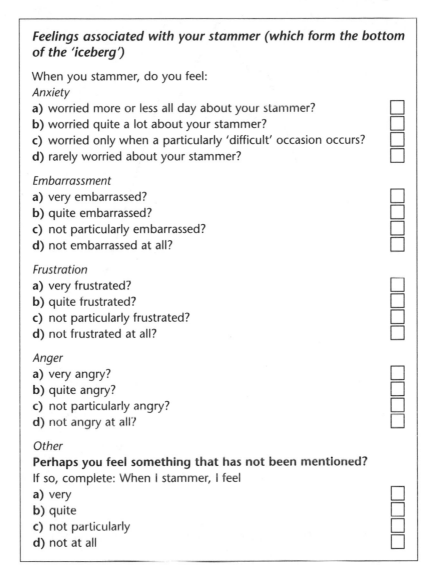

Feelings associated with your stammer (which form the bottom of the 'iceberg')

When you stammer, do you feel:

Anxiety
a) worried more or less all day about your stammer? ☐
b) worried quite a lot about your stammer? ☐
c) worried only when a particularly 'difficult' occasion occurs? ☐
d) rarely worried about your stammer? ☐

Embarrassment
a) very embarrassed? ☐
b) quite embarrassed? ☐
c) not particularly embarrassed? ☐
d) not embarrassed at all? ☐

Frustration
a) very frustrated? ☐
b) quite frustrated? ☐
c) not particularly frustrated? ☐
d) not frustrated at all? ☐

Anger
a) very angry? ☐
b) quite angry? ☐
c) not particularly angry? ☐
d) not angry at all? ☐

Other
Perhaps you feel something that has not been mentioned?
If so, complete: When I stammer, I feel
a) very ☐
b) quite ☐
c) not particularly ☐
d) not at all ☐

tive feelings about speech (bottom of the iceberg)? Or, perhaps, both aspects are significant in fairly equal proportions?

What does your iceberg look like?

Where are you going to draw your 'waterline' (Figure 6.2)?

As you look at your iceberg, where have you put the dividing line? What ratio do you have between the overt stammer and the covert feel-

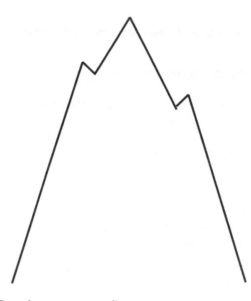

Figure 6.2   Drawing your waterline

ings? Do you perceive your difficulty as being mainly concerned with speech, and so your iceberg looks somewhat like Mala's? Or have you come to the decision that, like Josh, your predicament has as much, or more, to do with your negative feelings?

Did you know in advance what your iceberg would look like or are you surprised?

Whatever your iceberg looks like and whatever your answer to these questions, you have now made a definite start in getting a clearer picture, and a greater understanding of your personal stammering situation.

Main points in this chapter

You are invited to construct you own 'iceberg' by considering:
- How you stammer.
- How you feel when you stammer.

7

More about your stammer

In the last chapter you were invited to look at your core stammering behaviours and at associated feelings. In this chapter, we would like you to consider some other relevant aspects – in particular, your 'secondary behaviours'.

Secondary behaviours are the coping strategies used by all adults who stammer in order to avoid the moment of stammering, to escape from the unpleasant sensation of the stammer, or to get speech started. Unlike the core behaviours, these are not basic, involuntary actions. The secondary behaviours are built up gradually over time; they are acquired as learnt reactions to the core difficulty and then become an integral part of the individual's stammering pattern.

The secondary behaviours include:

Avoidance

It is useful to consider how hard you try to avoid your stammer and, therefore, the degree to which you need to hide it. If you have a severe, frequent stammer, you may be unable or unwilling to hide it; in which case, the people you know, and those that you meet, will be aware of how you speak. If you have a job, then your employer will know that you stammer; if you have a partner, your partner will know and, if you are at college, your tutors will know. Although you may well be anxious, you will probably not be in a state approaching panic because you have allowed others to hear you and you are out in the open – overt. Conversely, if your stammer is mild and infrequent, you can spend a considerable amount of energy in avoiding being heard to stammer so that your employer and close friends may be unaware. In this scenario you have set up a 'persona' as a fluent speaker, and so your anxiety and fear of being 'found out' can be extremely high. You could find it hard and painful to admit to yourself how much you avoid and hide, but we hope the following explanations and questions will be helpful.

Avoidance can occur at different levels:

Avoiding words

Craig had to buy a train ticket to Waterloo Station every few weeks. He was convinced that he could not say 'Waterloo' because 'w' was a difficult sound for him. He acquired an avoidance trick. This entailed him going up to the ticket counter, and then pretending to have a coughing fit. During this 'coughing fit', he would pull a used ticket out of his pocket and point to the word 'Waterloo' – and thus obtain his ticket.

Avoiding situations

Bina had stammered for as long as she could remember, and her great fear was public speaking. She managed to avoid this all her life, but now had a new job and found that she was required to give a presentation. Bina worried and worried about this and, eventually, phoned in sick on the morning of the presentation.

Avoidance strategies

1 **Avoiding being heard**
   How do you avoid being heard stammering?
   I give up when I have difficulty
   I substitute words
   I change the order of words
   I pretend to be thinking about what I want to say
   I stop talking when I would like to say more
   I don't talk
   I try to keep talking without pausing to take a breath
   I split up words, i.e. break up one-syllable words into two syllables
   I begin to speak when someone else is talking
   Something other than the above

2 **Postponing or putting off the moment of stammering**
   How do you postpone?
   I pause
   I beat around the bush
   I repeat previous words or phrases (take a run up to a hard word)
   I introduce unnecessary sounds before a difficult word
   I pretend not to hear
   I start again and again until the message becomes muddled
   Something other than the above

Avoiding accepting the stammer

David is 32 and has stammered since the age of about three. While at primary school, he remembers an adult telling him that he would 'grow out of it'. He has clung to this thought all his life and, although he knows that he stammers, he does not accept the situation. He continues to believe that he will 'grow out of it' – his feeling is that the stammer is like having a cold, and that he will wake up one morning and find that it has gone. At his age, this is not realistic.

Avoiding talking about the stammer

Luke is 15. He has a mild to moderate stammer and manages to hide it on most occasions by various strategies that he uses. He is very ashamed of, and embarrassed by, his speech difficulty and has never spoken about it to anyone – not his parents, teachers, siblings or friends.

---

3 Using 'starters' or tactics to get speech going

How do you get speech started when you are blocked by a stammer?

Shift my body	Jerk my head
Clear my throat	Tap my foot
Snap my fingers	Move my hand/hands
Lick my lips	Click my tongue
Talk higher or lower	Speak louder or softer
Speak faster or slower	Other than the above
Yawn	

4 Acceptance

Do you know that you stammer but do not accept yourself as a stammerer or person who stammers?

a) I never accept myself as a stammerer ☐
b) Most of the time, I do not accept myself as a stammerer ☐
c) Most of the time, I accept myself as a stammerer ☐
d) I always accept myself as a stammerer ☐

5 Talking about your stammer with other people

Do you talk about your stammer with other people?

a) never ☐
b) very rarely ☐
c) most of the time ☐
d) all the time ☐

At this stage, you might want to look at your own secondary behaviours. The list in the box on the previous pages provides some strategies that are frequently used to cope with stammering. Tick the ones that you use.

None of the behaviours listed under avoidance strategies are necessary in order to talk – all the behaviours are *learnt* and have developed around the stammer.

If you have ticked mainly (a) answers, this suggests that you are extremely worried about what people will think if they know about your speech and that you do everything you can to hide it; (b) answers show that you still use a considerable amount of avoidance; (c) answers suggest you are fairly open about your stammer, and (d) responses indicate that you talk about your stammer and allow people to hear it, and you will probably *not* have a high anxiety level.

You could think of your stammer as being like an onion which has many layers, and only the central part is the core behaviour; all the layers are secondary, acquired behaviours.

Figure 7.1 is the 'onion' that was drawn by Keith (age 59).

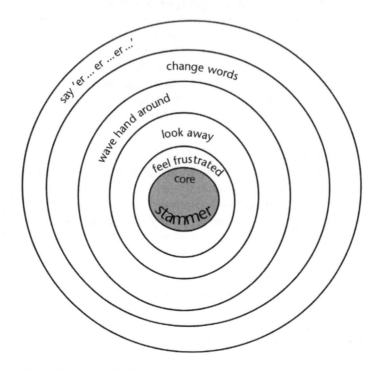

Figure 7.1 The stammering 'onion'

Other associated speech behaviours

Speech behaviours

How fast do you speak?
a) very fast
b) sometimes very fast
c) average rate
d) quite slowly

How much fluency do you have?
a) approximately 25%
b) approximately 55%
c) approximately 75%
d) approximately 95%

How tense are you?
a) I am tense most of the time
b) I am a fairly tense person
c) I am only tense when I stammer
d) I am rarely, if ever, tense

Speech rate

Some people are naturally fast talkers so that, whereas the average rate of speech is about 120–160 words per minute, a fast speaker can be at 200 words per minute or more. Speech rate is an important issue in stammering because someone who stammers may:

- talk more quickly in order to hide the stammer;
- talk too quickly and aggravate the stammer;
- increase the speech rate just before and after a stammer;
- feel that there is a need to rush through speech in order to avoid irritating or boring the listener.

Fluency

The stammer can be so powerful that, although many people, such as Josh, report that 70–90 per cent of their speech is fluent, it is easy to overlook your own fluency. If your answer is in the (c) or (d) section in the exercise above, then you have a large amount of fluent speech and need to examine whether you notice, and value, your natural fluency.

Tension

Tension is always an issue in adult stammering, but how big an issue depends on the individual speaker; (a) or (b) responses in the exercise in the above box would suggest that you see yourself as quite a tense person most of the time, while a (c) answer means you feel tense only when stammering; a (d) response implies that you view yourself as a relaxed person.

These findings have obvious implications for the therapy that would be likely to help you; for example, a very tense person would need more therapy or self-help on that aspect than someone who felt very relaxed.

There is one further area of enquiry that may be useful and that is:

Thoughts and feelings

Thoughts may sometimes appear to overlap with feelings, but there is a difference. Most of us have experienced situations where we think that we were really good at something and yet felt that we could not do whatever it was. For example:

'I know I am good at exams, but I *feel* that I am going to fail all the time.'
'I had an excellent appraisal at work, but I always *feel* that I will get the sack.'
'I know I have a good social life, but I often *feel* that people don't like me.'
'I know I am looking good tonight, but I *feel* unattractive.'

And then, of course:

'I know my friends don't judge me by my stammer, but I *feel* that they do.'

How thoughts influence feelings

We have mentioned previously that your thoughts can influence your feelings; for example, Mary gets up in the morning, sees that it is pouring with rain and thinks, 'Good, it's raining so I won't need to water the garden.' This positive thought about a grey, miserable day makes her feel happy and to look forward to the day. John gets up on the same morning, he sees the same pouring rain and thinks, 'Oh no, it's raining so I won't be able to paint the fence.' His negative thoughts make him feel annoyed and predict a miserable and boring day.

Mary and John have seen the same rain on the same morning, but their different thoughts affect the way they both feel about the day ahead. In the same way, someone who stammers can go into a shop, ask for an item, and see the assistant smile. The response to the smile could be 'What a cheerful, friendly girl' or 'She has heard the stammer and thinks it sounds stupid'.

Whatever you think about an incident affects the way you feel about it.

The questions in the exercise box below are aimed at this issue because they are concerned with a range of thoughts from positive to negative, and those thoughts will affect your feelings. Tick the boxes applicable to you.

Thoughts related to my stammer

Concern about what other people think
a) I worry all the time about what others think of me ☐
b) I worry quite a lot ☐
c) I am not particularly concerned ☐
d) I hardly, if ever, worry about what people think of me ☐

How much my stammer affects me
a) it dominates my life ☐
b) it's a nuisance – but I can live with it ☐
c) not much – only on specific occasions,
   e.g. presentations, interviews, etc. ☐
d) very rarely, if at all ☐

How much my stammer has held me back at work/school
a) very much ☐
b) quite a lot ☐
c) occasionally – a little ☐
d) rarely, if ever ☐

How much my stammer has held me back socially
a) very much ☐
b) quite a lot ☐
c) occasionally – a little ☐
d) rarely, if ever ☐

If your answers are mainly (a) you are probably very concerned about what other people think of you; your thoughts tend to be negative about people's reactions to your speech, and you feel that you are seriously disadvantaged at work and/or socially. Mostly (b) answers imply you have some of the same beliefs and thoughts as do people in the (a) group, but do not feel as strongly about these issues. Mainly (c) responses indicate that what others think is not of vital importance to you and, although you feel that you are occasionally disadvantaged at work/school and/or socially, this is not a central issue. Mainly (d) answers show that what others think is of little importance to you and you do not feel disadvantaged by your stammer.

What have you discovered in this chapter?

The main things I have learnt about my secondary stammering behaviours are:

The main things that I do to hide/avoid/postpone my stammer are:

The main thoughts that affect my feelings are:

You now have the following:
- An iceberg showing the ratio between your overt core stammering behaviours and the covert feelings.
- An onion representing certain strategies you have acquired over the years to avoid a stammer, and some of your feelings about stammering.

Main points in this chapter

- The secondary behaviours that have become associated with the stammer over the years.
- Avoidance, postponement and starters.
- Other speech behaviours.
- Concerns about what people think about you and your speech.
- Fluency.
- Drawing your own stammering 'onion'.
- Your thoughts and attitudes about stammering.

8

The mechanics of speech and stammering

Now that you have a clearer idea about your stammer, what can you do about it? It is always best to seek the help of a registered speech and language therapist (SLT). If you live in the UK, the British Stammering Association (BSA) has a list of NHS speech and language therapists specializing in the treatment of stammering. If you live in another country, you will find the names and addresses of other associations in Useful addresses at the back of this book. You may also wish to investigate alternative help available in your area. We would like to reiterate that this book is not written as a substitute for professional help, but rather to augment such help, or to assist if you are unable to access professional support.

Many people who stammer have found it useful to consider how speech is produced so that some of the reasons for the occurrence of

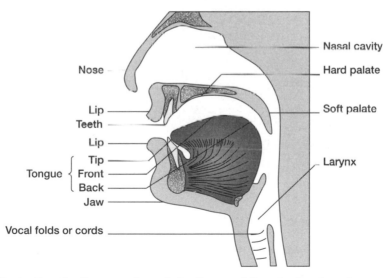

Illustration 1 Cross-section of the face and throat, showing the speech organs

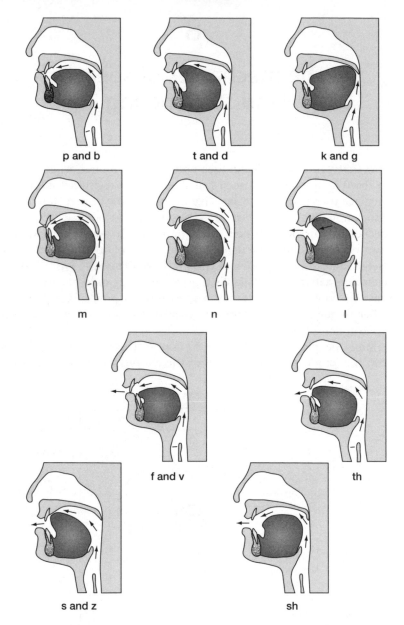

Illustration 2   Position of the speech organs during the production of consonant sounds

blocks can be explained. Without this knowledge, the whole issue of stammering can seem mysterious and inaccessible, and this leads to feelings of helplessness in dealing with it.

How sounds are made

Air is breathed in through the nose and mouth and goes into the lungs (Illustration 1). It is then exhaled and passes through the vocal cords, also called vocal folds or voice box, which are contained in the larynx (at the level of the Adam's apple). If the vocal cords vibrate, then voice is produced; if no vibration occurs, then the air continues silently through the throat and into the mouth.

The different sounds of speech are produced by modification of the air stream through a variety of movements of the speech organs – lips, teeth, tongue, palate and jaw. Consonant sounds are formed because two speech organs touch, or nearly touch (see Illustration 2), while all the vowel sounds – a, e, i, o, u – are voiced and, therefore, the vocal cords must vibrate.

The consonant sounds tend to go in pairs – for example, p and b, s and z. In order to make the pair of sounds, the movement of the speech organs is identical, but one of the pair requires vibration of the cords because voice is needed, whereas the other has no vocal cord vibration and so it is voiceless. For example, to make a p or b sound, you need to get your lips together and open them again, allowing some air to explode out. Although the movement is the same, the p and b sounds are different – in order to say b, the cords need to vibrate and produce voice; to say the p sound, you just need air coming through the open vocal cords, into the mouth and to the lips (be careful that you do not add a vowel and say 'puh' or 'pa').

Look at Figure 8.1.

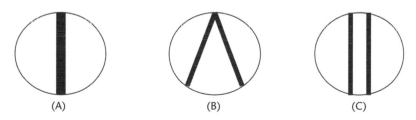

(A)   (B)   (C)

Figure 8.1   A view of the larynx containing vocal cords looking down from the mouth

To experience tightly closed cords, cough gently because, during the cough, your cords will be in position (A).

Breathe out gently and your cords will be in the open position (B).

Hum gently and put your hand on, or in the area of, your Adam's apple. Can you feel the vibration of (C)?

Experiment for yourself by doing the following

Make some sounds and work out how you make each sound – which of the speech organs is moving? Notice how the breath is released – does it explode out suddenly or flow out smoothly? Discover whether there is vibration of the cords – are you more tense for some sounds than for others? Which of the speech organs moves when you say the following single sounds?

t (as in tea)

m (as in more)

ee (as in meet)

ah, oo, and ee – can you feel the vibration for these voiced sounds when you put your hand on your throat?

s, f and k – these are sounds that require no vibration as they are voiceless – can you feel the difference?

s then z – feel how the vibration only happens on the z sound. In that pair, s is voiceless and z has voice.

Think of a word on which you tend to block. Now replicate that block as closely as you can and, while doing this, try to feel what is happening to your:

lips, tongue, area round the mouth and throat?
vocal cords – is there vibration or not?
tension – if so, where?
sensations other than the above?

What have you discovered from the above exercise?

When speaking, we use words and sentences – not single sounds. Unless there is a block, we are largely unaware of the production of individual sounds because the movements of the speech organs are extremely rapid in order to move from sound to sound to make words and sentences. It is necessary for the speech organs to move quickly and with accuracy in order to produce a smooth flow of speech and, at the same time, the cords must vibrate or stay open depending on the sounds that are being made.

Why do I block and 'get stuck'?

It is possible to repeat or prolong sounds and syllables without unnecessary muscular tension, but it is impossible to block unless there is excessive tension in some part of the vocal mechanism.

Read the following phrase: I SAT DOWN.

We say that phrase in one go, on one breath stream. Now let us examine the word 'I', which is a vowel, needs voice and, therefore, vibration of the cords, but the next word 'sat' starts and ends with voiceless sounds – s and t.

Apart from all the movements required to make those sounds, within a split second, we now need to have no vibration of the cords for s, vibration of the cords for a, and no vibration for t.

Fluent speech requires amazingly rapid co-ordination of muscles and breath flow. Thinking of it in that way, it seems remarkable that we can speak at all. The good news is that we can do so because all these movements become automatic and are acquired in early childhood. French children speak French, Chinese children speak Chinese, English children speak English. It is also interesting to consider that the majority of people throughout the world speak more than one language!

If for some reason tension creeps into any part of the vocal tract and prevents the quick, precise muscular movements required for smooth speech, then a block can ensue. Most stammers occur at the beginning of words and, especially, at the beginning of a conversation – it is a bit like starting a car from cold.

If a word starts with a voiced sound and there is tension, the vocal cords can close in a block, and it is then impossible to achieve the vibration necessary to produce that voiced sound. If the word starts with a voiceless sound, it will almost always be followed by a voiced sound – for example, s-a-t, f-o-r or s-o-n-g, and so on. Stammerers may find it difficult to make the quick transition from voiceless to voiced because any tension in the cords will make it hard to move smoothly from no vibration to vibration, and back again.

Main points in this chapter

- How speech sounds are made.
- The vocal cords and voiced and voiceless sounds.
- An outline of the main reasons for blocks, tense repetitions and prolongations.
- Tension in the vocal cords or folds.

9

Theories and therapies

We can now return to the 'icebergs' of stammering (Chapter 1). Look at Figure 9.1.

Looking at these icebergs, it will be apparent that there is a wide range of possible combinations of overt speech behaviours and covert hidden feelings. Moreover, we are not discussing icebergs floating in a stormy sea, but the speech difficulties of adults who have widely different backgrounds, ethnic origins, life experiences, abilities, loves, hates and aims. When we consider these factors, it becomes evident that not every type of therapy is suitable for each person who stammers. Many speech and language therapists believe that a flexible approach is needed to deal with this diversity.

There are exceptions to most rules, but, generally, the more severe the stammer, the less you may want help with covert aspects. This is because if you have a considerable struggle getting the words out, then initially you will probably want a fluency technique to make life easier for you. Conversely, the milder the stammer, and the more interiorized or hidden that it is, the greater the anxieties and the more you may want to get help with sorting out your uncomfortable feelings about speech, and the fear of being heard to stammer.

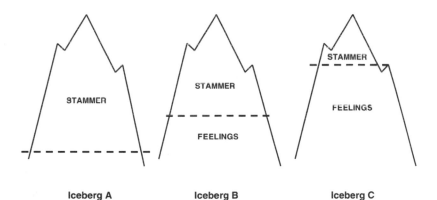

Figure 9.1   The stammering 'icebergs'

When studying Chapter 8 on the mechanics of speech production, it is clear that to produce smooth, easy speech, we need to co-ordinate a sufficiently relaxed speech mechanism with adequate breath control, with the production of voice when required, and with the precise muscular movements necessary to construct the sounds that make up words. For this reason, many forms of therapy, especially those aimed at fluency, will encourage work on breath control, voice (vocal) production and easy articulation. The variety of fluency-enhancing therapy methods occur because of the differing importance that is placed on one or more of these aspects – some methods put considerable stress on breath control, some emphasize voice production, and others consider soft articulation to be of fundamental importance.

The present situation

Over the years, two schools of thought have emerged about the treatment of adult stammering. In the mid-twentieth century, Professor Charles Van Riper, a lifelong stammerer, developed a treatment approach based on his own experiences, and on his knowledge as a professor of audiology and speech pathology. This method deals with the overt and covert aspects and is called stammering modification. Later that century, another approach evolved that dealt more with the physical or mechanical side of speech. Therapists and clients alike were sometimes confused by which approach to use and the situation was clarified when, in 1979, Professor Hugo Gregory (also a lifelong stammerer) described these two methods in his book called *Controversies about Stuttering Therapy*. He called the two approaches 'Stammer more Easily' and 'Speak more Fluently'.[2]

The 'Stammer more Easily' method

The 'Stammer more Easily' methods are loosely based on the works of Charles Van Riper and of Joseph Sheehan, who were both university professors who stammered, and who both spent a considerable part of their lives researching stammering, and working with people who stammered. The 'Stammer more Easily' methods have as their main aim to help you to modify both the stammer and the associated negative feelings and attitudes, and to reduce the amount of avoidance strategies. The reasoning is, as an adult, you come to therapy with a stammer that comprises both overt and covert aspects. You may also have a considerable amount of natural fluency. A fluency technique alone does not address the whole difficulty. Therefore, it is advisable to help you to take control of the stammer when it occurs and, by modifying and reducing the struggle and tension, as well as the negative feelings and unrealistic attitudes, you can learn to take charge of your speech, rather than allowing the speech to be in charge of you.

There are several techniques used in this approach and they include the following:

Identification

You are asked to analyse both covert and overt aspects of your individual way of stammering. This stage helps you to formulate a profile of what you do, and what you feel. Once you have identified these issues, you have a stable base from which to tackle your speech.

Desensitization

Most adults are sensitive about being heard to stammer – especially in situations when they think that fluency is necessary, or when they especially want to impress. This sensitivity can cause excessive attention to the stammer, and create undue tension because energy is wasted on the struggle to appear fluent. During the desensitization programme, negative thoughts and attitudes are examined and discussed, and carefully graded steps are designed to help you to be more open about your stammer, and to face some of your feared situations. These, and other strategies, are geared to help develop less sensitivity and, with a change of attitude, to have more energy to deal with the actual speech difficulty.

Reducing avoidance strategies

The moment of stammering is frequently avoided and the result is that this vital moment is never, or rarely, experienced. Unfortunately, avoidance may give temporary relief but, in the long term, the more you avoid, the more you have to avoid because avoidance increases fear. In order to move forward, it is necessary to work on your avoidance 'tricks', and learn new techniques that will help you to cope with the stammer instead of running away from it. If, like many others, you have used a whole raft of avoidance strategies in the past, this can be a demanding stage in the therapy programme. As with other techniques, it may well prove a surprisingly liberating and satisfying experience.

Accepting your stammer instead of fighting it

Acknowledging to yourself, and later to others, that you have a stammer is an important step. You will be helped to consider that your stammer is not a life-threatening problem, that it is nothing to be ashamed of, that you have many assets and skills, and that your speech is only a small part of you as a whole person. Accepting the situation will help you to deal with it and move forward.

Stammering more easily

Learning new ways of coping with the physical aspects is also incorporated in this method. Various techniques are employed to deal with the muscular movements of the speech and vocal mechanism, reduce tension and deal with the stammer at the moment that it occurs. Many of the techniques used in this stage are similar to those of the 'Speak more Fluently' approach.

The 'Speak more Fluently' method

The 'Speak more Fluently' methods are now frequently called 'fluency shaping', and these techniques deal essentially with the physical side of speaking. They have as their main aim helping you to become more fluent by retraining the speech and vocal muscles to move more smoothly and easily. The reasoning is that you come to therapy to become more fluent and, therefore, help must be directed towards teaching a more fluent way of speaking. When fluency is achieved, the fears and anxieties previously related to the stammer may well diminish, and attitudes to speaking will probably change.

It must be emphasized that there are no magic cures, and all the techniques taught in this approach require daily, continuous practice for quite a period of time.

Among the techniques used are:

1 Slowing down the rate of speech. It has been found that doing no more than slowing down the rate can make a noticeable difference to the stammer. This is due to several aspects linked to giving yourself more time to:
   - reduce the feelings of urgency and haste;
   - develop awareness and control of speech elements that are otherwise too fast to notice or control;
   - decrease tension;
   - think about how to manage your speech;
   - think about precisely what you want to say;
   - breathe;
   - calm down.

2 Relaxed breathing. Many programmes incorporate breathing, or focus solely on it, because:
   - When breathing is relaxed, it will relax not only your whole body,

but your throat, the vocal folds, lips, tongue and jaw so that the speech musculature is as free from tension as possible.

- Under stress, you may try too hard to talk, causing undue tension in the vocal folds; air then becomes trapped between the lungs and the throat and cannot escape, and the result is that you are literally holding your breath. This causes feelings of breathlessness.
- Speech is based on breathing. Without breath we cannot live, but with tense, fragmented breathing we can cause, or exacerbate, stammering.

Breathing exercises may concentrate on diaphragmatic or thoracic breathing, or a mixture of both of these methods.

3 Vocal fold management. This is also called voice production. Your vocal folds are flaps of muscle in your throat at the level of the Adam's apple. If you hum gently and place your fingers on your throat, you can feel the folds vibrating. In Chapter 8, on normal speech production, we noted that in English, and indeed all languages, there are both voiced and voiceless sounds. The relaxed movement of the vocal folds is essential for the smooth transition from voiced to voiceless and vice versa; blocks occur when tension in the folds makes it impossible for vibration to occur and then voice cannot be produced. Techniques are taught that increase awareness of the vocal folds and facilitate sufficient movement. Among other techniques, prolongation or stretching of the vowel sounds and the voiced consonants (m, n, l, r, v, z) is sometimes encouraged because, during prolongation, there is continuous vibration of the folds.

4 Soft contacts. This is also called gentle onset. The contact of the speech organs that is required to make the consonant sounds of speech is described in Chapter 8. When blocks occur, there is excessive tension and the muscles required to make the necessary contacts are too taut to move efficiently. For example, when trying to say 'today', in order to say the initial t sound, you need to lift the tip of the tongue to a position behind your upper teeth and then release the tongue to form the o sound that follows. When there is too much tension in the tongue, the release does not occur and speakers complain that their tongue 'gets stuck'. The work on acquiring this skill will help you to keep the speech organs sufficiently relaxed so that gentle and light contacts can be achieved instead of the hard contacts that occur when stammering.

A large number of therapy methods?

The idea that there is an almost infinite number of ways of dealing with stammering causes unnecessary confusion because:

- Almost all forms of therapy can be grouped under Gregory's two main headings.
- There is a variety of methods classified under each heading – after all, the training programme for the English football team will not be identical to that from Brazil, but the main aim for both teams is to win the next match.
- Practitioners use slightly different ways of applying procedures – think back to your school days. Most of us can remember various different teaching methods, but the main aim was to get us to learn a specific subject.

Gregory's two central methods are not mutually exclusive because it has been found that, when using a fluency shaping technique alone, the old feelings of anxiety and fear do not necessarily go away, even when you become more fluent, and so, for some people, the changes in fluency tend to be temporary. There are mix-and-match or integrated procedures when the therapist concentrates mainly on one of the above approaches, but also introduces aspects of the other. Most adults will need to address both the stammer and the feelings, but you have to discover which is your most important speech issue at this time, while the therapist needs to consider every client as an individual and vary the importance placed on each approach accordingly.

Karen

Karen is 27 years old. She is married with two small children and has stammered ever since she can remember. She has had various forms of therapy over the years and has summed up the situation as follows:

'I have learnt that stammering therapy is not one thing or something that you do once and that's it. It is a process, a progression that moves with you as you go on with your life. When I was 16, I just wanted to be fluent and so I worked at a fluency shaping technique. I still use that technique sometimes, but I have changed. When I trained and qualified as a nurse, I got very anxious in case I couldn't tell relatives about a patient or I got mixed up when giving information to a doctor. I went back to therapy and learnt a lot about negative feelings and positive self-talk and attitude change.

'Now I'm married and have kids – I'm still the same person but my priorities have altered – my outlook has changed and so has my stammer. The stammer isn't very bad any more and I don't think about it as being an important part of my life, like I did when I was 16. Me and my stammer are at a different stage in life and I realize that I have gone through a process of changing both my speech and my attitude. Some of the changes were due to therapy, but some are due to me and the changes in my life.'

You may be reading this book because you have no access to speech and language therapy or any other help, and so we will be including some self-help advice in Chapters 10 and 11. If there is help available to you, the range of therapies on offer will depend on where you live, whether there are specialist centres, and the service provisions made locally. The BSA has a list of UK therapists specializing in the treatment of stammering, and it is advisable to contact the BSA and discover what is available in your area. Many other countries have associations that you can locate through a website provided in Useful addresses.

You may feel, 'What is the point of describing the range of therapeutic procedures and the types of therapy when I will have little chance of getting the help that I decide I need?' We would reiterate that nearly all the therapies come under two main headings and so, if there is a service where you live, you will have every chance of getting the help that you need – it is only the specific method or the range of procedures that may differ from one area to another.

Main points in this chapter

- People differ in what they want from therapy.
- There is no one-size-fits-all method.
- 'Stammer more Easily' and 'Speak more Fluently' are the headings under which therapies can be grouped.
- Integrated approaches.

10

Self-help – general aspects

This chapter contains some initial advice, principles and exercises that will be of use to most teenagers and adults who stammer, whatever their 'iceberg' of stammering. More specific exercises, focused on overt and covert aspects, are included in Chapter 11.

Be your own therapist

If you are working on your own, you have no choice because you need to become your own therapist. If you are presently working with a therapist, you will eventually have to cope by yourself. What do you require to be your own therapist so that you can help yourself effectively?

- Information – we hope this book will give you an adequate amount.
- Be honest with yourself about where and when you tend to stammer, and what you feel about stammering.
- Consider carefully the exercise or exercises that will help you.
- Use the exercises in this chapter as a starting point and be inventive about setting yourself graded tasks to extend your work on a given item.
- Accept the fact that you have had years of practising stammering, so you now need to practise regularly, and for a considerable time, to replace the stammer with a different way of speaking.
- You may not be able to be fluent all the time, but step by step you can make vast improvements in your speaking.
- You have had years of avoiding words and situations so that your negative thoughts and feelings are well established.
- You can improve your feelings about speaking and about yourself as a speaker.

We have divided the self-help chapters into three sections:

- General (Section 1)
- Increasing fluency, and stammering more easily (Section 2)
- Avoidance, feelings and attitudes (Section 3).

Section 1 is in this chapter and Sections 2 and 3 are in the following one (Chapter 11). The sections are not mutually exclusive and, inevitably, there is overlap between them.

We suggest that you:

- refer to your 'iceberg' in Chapters 6 and 7 to help in establishing the items that are specific to your stammering difficulties;
- choose whatever is applicable to you and ignore the rest. There is a wide choice in order to cover most people's needs;
- begin with an option that is easy for you rather than the one you feel you 'should' push yourself to do;
- concentrate on one item at a time and work with it until you feel comfortable.

(Please note that although Appendix C is concerned with slowing down the rate of speech, it may be useful for other work because it outlines a graded exercise plan.)

Section 1 – General

Change

Tackling your stammer will inevitably involve change, whether that be change of speech, feelings, thoughts or all of these. The reason change has to occur is because if you keep on doing what you are doing now, then the results will continue to be exactly as they are now. If you continue to think, 'I'm not going to be able to say my name without getting completely stuck', then this will lead to feelings of anxiety, your

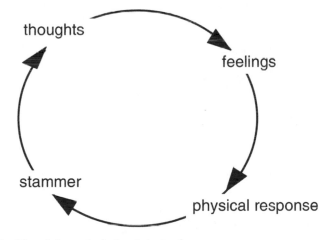

Figure 10.1 The vicious circle in stammering

physical response could be tension, followed by the actual behaviour – which in this case is stammering (see Figure 10.1). In order to break this vicious circle, some change must occur, and that change will take time.

Start by making yourself a hierarchy or ladder

The purpose of constructing your own hierarchy or ladder is to work out the speaking situations that you consider 'easy' and those that you believe are 'difficult'. You can then move slowly, step by step, up the ladder. In our example there are 10 steps, but the number of steps you choose is up to you.

For most people the ease or difficulty of a speaking situation is related to:

- the supposed threat or stress caused by a listener(s). You may have no difficulty saying 'Good morning' to your friend, but find it hard to say 'Good morning' to your boss or head teacher;
- the content or importance of what you are saying – when you talk about something vague and rather unimportant like the weather, your speech will probably be easier than when you have to do a presentation, describe something in detail, or give important information.

When undertaking self-help work, it is prudent to consider both the listener or listeners, and the content of what you are saying. In order to practise effectively, use your personal hierarchy. It makes sense to start with the easiest situations and work slowly up that ladder, because starting with the most difficult one is unlikely to prove successful in the long run.

In the box below we have listed ten speaking situations as an example:

Most difficult

10 In a meeting of heads of departments.
9 When giving a presentation.
8 In the pub if it's very crowded and I have to shout.
7 With my line manager.
6 With a group of people at work.
5 Asking for something complicated in a shop.
4 With my mother.
3 With my friend Brian.
2 With Brian's three-year-old child.
1 With my dog.

Easiest

Slowing down

What do you think helps you to achieve more fluency? The answer to this question is frequently, 'I need to speak more slowly'. You may already have instinctively, or deliberately, slowed down your rate of speaking and found this helpful. There may be other ways that you have coped, but some of these, such as avoiding words and situations, are not useful in the long run.

Slowing down the rate of speech is an almost universal aid, but solely slowing down your speech may be hard if you are rushing around every moment of the day. It is helpful to look at several aspects of slowing down:

1 Slowing down generally if life is one long rush.
2 Slowing down by resisting time pressure both in everyday life and in your speech.
3 Slowing down the rate of speech.
4 Using pauses rather than hurrying on with speech.
5 Slowing down the actual moment of stammering.

1 Slowing down generally Give some careful thought as to whether you could find one or two occasions every day to deliberately take your life at a slower pace. This can greatly reduce feelings of anxiety and help with your speech. Perhaps you could get up ten minutes earlier? Go for a walk in the lunch hour? Wait to open your emails? Make a list and prioritize? Learn to say 'No'? You will be able to think of ways that suit your lifestyle.

2 Time pressure Do you think that you, and your speech, are under time pressure and that this is imposed on you either by others or by yourself? Do you feel any of the following?

● Dread of pauses or silence because of fear that you will be unable to start speaking again.
● Everything goes quiet when you begin to speak.
● You are not entitled to take up the listener's time, or that you are boring.
● You must speak faster and faster (increased rate causes increased struggle).
● Anxiety increases with authoritarian figures, groups and on the telephone.

Time pressure and feelings of urgency undoubtedly exacerbate stammering. The suggested approach is to become aware of when and why you find yourself under time pressure, and also to identify how much of this pressure comes from you. Thereafter, you can decide in which situations you deliberately choose to resist this pressure. You can find further advice in the item on Pausing later in this section.

Suggested exercises

- Collect seven instances of time pressure. Try to work out how much of the pressure you felt was due to the other person's behaviour and how much was your own, internalized time pressure.
- Note at least five words on which you hurry yourself just to get the words over and done with as quickly as possible.
- Collect five situations in which you feel time pressure is imposed on you and you are able to resist/not able to resist. Telephone operators, shop assistants, bus drivers and bar staff all do an outstanding job of creating time pressure! Perhaps your line manager, or someone else at work, does an equally good job?
- Collect five situations in which you put pressure on yourself. One of the words most frequently hurried is 'hello'.
- Choose the 'easiest' situation on your hierarchy and deliberately slow down your rate of speech and increase your pausing for a sentence or two. Note how the listener reacts (if at all) and how you feel.

---

3 Slowing down the rate of speech   It has been found that slowing down the rate of speech will in itself reduce the frequency and severity of stammering. There is no suggestion that you should speak abnormally slowly, but rather that you consider slowing down your normal rate in order to gain more control.

You might like to experiment with slowing down the rate at which you speak and, if successful, continue with this approach.

Some people, both fluent and stammering, find slowing down difficult to achieve and, in that case, there is a programme of work that can be followed in Appendix C. Whether or not you decide to work on slowing down, the programme in Appendix C could be useful to illustrate a step-by-step approach that you can adapt to other items.

When slowing down your speech, be aware of the most common mistakes made so that you can avoid these:

- Jumping from word to word so that, although the speech is slowed down, it is jerky and lacking in smoothness.

- Getting so focused on slowing down that you forget to pause.
- Taking very deep breaths as though about to go deep-sea diving.

A tape recorder, recording CD player, mobile phone or other recording method will be helpful to keep information on your practice, and to check your work. If you cannot record, just make sure that you do not rush through this work by going straight for your most difficult situation. Whichever item in this chapter you choose to practise, your foundations must be solid.

While working on slowing down, use your hierarchy:

- Start by working on your own (no listener) until you feel comfortable, then move to:
- One close friend or relative (friendly, easy listener).
- Gradually work your way to the more difficult listeners in your life.

At the same time:

- Build the content of your speech in easy stages.
- Start with reading (the words are provided, it is not emotional, you can concentrate on the technique – your slower way of talking).
- Then move to talking by yourself – monologue (find a private place and just begin to talk using the technique).

When you feel secure reading and talking by yourself, you are ready to use your slower way of talking in short conversations.

You can either practise reading a short passage from a book or newspaper at a fairly slow rate (if you have a stopwatch, aim for 60–80 words per minute) or, if you prefer, turn to Appendix C where there is some graded reading.

You may find that reading out loud by yourself is an easy task and that you hardly, if ever, stammer, so it may seem as if this form of practice is a waste of time. Not so. The purpose of this work is for you to find a level of speech where you can maintain fluency, and become aware of how you can change your speech in order to create that fluency. It is absolutely not a test of how often you can stammer! Conversely, if you find that you stammer a great deal while reading, then you are not going slowly enough for your facility, and you will need to slow down a little more. Bear in mind that a very slow rate is for practice purposes only and not for everyday use.

If possible, practise twice a day for 5–10 minutes. Gradually bring your new way of talking into a conversation with someone who is easy on your hierarchy. One sentence at a time is enough to start with. Step by step, work up your ladder using your slower speech for longer periods, and in more difficult situations.

4 Using pauses It has been said that if there were only one piece of advice to give to someone who stammers, it should be to pause. Adults who stammer rarely have a normal pausing pattern because they think that, while they are speaking well, there is no point in stopping to pause because it might be difficult to start again, someone might interrupt, or a stammer will stop them soon enough.

The lack of pausing causes an abnormal rhythm to occur. Pausing is necessary to:

● breathe;
● think about what you want to say;
● think about how you want to say it;
● reduce rush and hurry;
● reduce anxiety;
● give the listener time to take in what you are saying;
● emphasize a point you are making (listen to politicians!);
● allow time to check your speech and reduce any tension that you find.

You could work on pausing straightaway, with the very next thing you say, and integrate it into the practice you do for slowing down. A good place to learn pausing is when answering a question. What do you do when someone asks 'What is your name?' Do you stop, pause, count to three, and then say, 'John Smith'? If you do that, congratulations, and you do not need to practise pausing; but if, when asked that question, you rush into the answer and often find that you are stammering, then this advice is for you. When someone asks you a question, *pause*, count to three silently, take a small breath in and, as you breathe out, give the answer. The result may surprise you.

5 Slow down your stammer It may sound quite a hard thing to do, but slowing down the actual moment when you stammer is a powerful tool because it can help you to feel more precisely what it is that you do at that moment. Try doing this in an easy situation. You might find that your instinct is to rush through the moment of stammering but, by slowing down, you get significant control over that moment and feel much more in charge of your speech.

Fluency

Stammering can be so powerful that the fluent periods are often ignored. Become aware of your fluency and value it. Be realistic and positive – most stammerers will have a considerable amount of fluency, but this is too often ignored. The fluent parts of your speech are just as important as the stammered parts. If you overlook your fluent speech, then you do not experience it – and this makes it difficult to extend the feelings, sensations and movements of the speech organs that occur during these periods.

Eye contact

Monitor your eye contact carefully so that you discover at what stage you look away or close your eyes – before, during or after the block or stammer? This action is part of your stammering behaviour and has developed over the years, either because you are embarrassed, or because you fear seeing an unsympathetic reaction. Your lack of comfortable eye contact with the listener tends to support and maintain the stammer, and increasing your eye contact will help you to feel more in control while stammering.

If you decide to do the following exercise, make sure that you keep your eye contact natural and that you do not stare at the listener. The following exercises can be done with people who are talking to you or to whom you are talking.

Eye contact

Days 1 and 2. Look at three people while they are talking to you. Are you really looking and listening? Do you feel comfortable looking at the speakers or are you staring at them?

Day 3. Write down the names of two people who are wearing glasses.

Day 4. Write down the names of two people who are wearing something black.

Day 5. Write down the names of three people who are talking very quickly.

Day 6. Write down the names of three people who have long hair.

Day 7. Write down the names of three people who have either good or bad eye contact while talking.

- Choose one of the easy situations on your hierarchy and make eye contact before a stammer occurs. Do this in easy situations for a week, perhaps two or three times per day.
- Now make eye contact before the stammer and maintain that eye contact during and immediately afterwards.
- Continue to observe the eye contact of other speakers and of yourself until you are comfortable with this exercise.

Listen to other speakers

Adults who stammer sometimes become so focused on their own speech that they cannot really listen to other speakers. Are you one of those who believe there are only two types of speakers – those who are fluent and those who stammer? If so, you are wrong. You may have got into the habit of thinking, 'Ann is so lucky. She talks all day, goes on and on, but she is always fluent.' Are you sure? When did you last really listen to Ann, or any other fluent speaker? It is important to listen attentively to other speakers partly because it helps to get a realistic picture of how others talk, and partly because it is of assistance in taking the focus off your own speech.

We are often told that the person presenting the news is very fluent, but that person is reading and we are discussing *talking*. The next time you are with so-called fluent speakers listen to how often they say 'um' and 'er', how often they hesitate while choosing the right word or thinking about what they want to say, or how often they go back and change something that they have said because they want to emphasize or correct. How fluent are they?

Of course, there is a difference between the not-fluent 'fluent' speaker and someone who stammers. One of the differences is that the so-called fluent speaker is not worried or anxious about common speech hesitations, while the person who stammers is highly concerned about any moment of non-fluency. It is essential to remember that no one, stammering or fluent, is ever 100 per cent fluent, so this is an unachievable goal – be sure not to aim for the impossible, but try to allow yourself to have some hesitancies while talking.

We hope that one or more items in this chapter will be helpful to you. There is more self-help in the next chapter.

Main points in this chapter

- Becoming your own therapist.
- Changing the vicious circle of stammering.
- Constructing a hierarchy or ladder.
- Slowing down.
- Pausing.
- Time pressure.
- Acknowledging your fluency.
- Increasing eye contact.
- Listening to the speech of others.

11

Self-help – overt and covert aspects

This chapter contains Sections 2 and 3 of the self-help guidelines. These sections are designed to be of assistance if you are unable to find professional help and wish to work on overt or covert aspects of your stammer. These aspects can be identified through using Chapters 6 and 7. Certain items contain short exercises, but extended exercises can be found in the Appendices at the end of the book.

Section 2 – Overt stammering

Increasing fluency

There are a number of techniques commonly used to increase fluency and modify moments of stammering, and they can be used if you have chosen to work on the overt part of your stammering 'iceberg'. You will probably have discovered some of these techniques for yourself – the most usual one is slowing down the rate of speech, as discussed in Chapter 10. Here are some more:

Breathe

'I feel out of breath' is heard frequently from people who stammer, and various forms of breathing difficulties do seem to occur. It is unclear whether these difficulties cause stammering or are due to the stammer. Whichever it is, co-ordinating breath with speech is essential and you may want to do some breath control work.

With all breathing exercises it is necessary to remain relaxed, check that your posture is good, and do not over-breathe. If you feel dizzy or faint, then you are over-breathing, so stop immediately.

The following is an exercise for expanding lung capacity and breath control:

- Breathe in. Make this a deep breath, but do not strain, keep relaxed, and make sure that your shoulders are down and that you do not over-breathe.
- Breathe out as slowly as possible, making a hissing noise on the sound sssssss.

- Work on this until you can hold the ssss for a comfortable length of time.
- Do this five times and twice a day if possible.
- Move to taking a breath in and, on the outgoing breath, count to 5.
- Do this exercise five times and twice a day if possible.
- Gradually, and when this suits you, on the outgoing breath count to 6, 7, and so on until you can comfortably reach 10 on one breath.
- After considerable practice, see how far you can count easily on one breath.

Further breathing exercises are given in Appendix D.

Vocal cord or vocal fold exercises

In a previous chapter, we have described how if the vocal cords close, then they cannot vibrate to produce voice, and that can lead to a block or tense repetition. It is helpful to work on increasing your awareness of vocal cord movements, and this is especially important for anyone whose speech contains tense, silent blocks.

Vocal exercises need a gentle, relaxed approach so that the voice is not pushed nor forced. Make sure that you breathe normally – neither taking an unusually deep breath nor gasping.

Try this short exercise:
Breathe in and, as you breathe out, make a gentle humming sound, like mmmmmmmmmm. Try to feel the vibration of your vocal cords. It may help to put your hand on the front of your throat at about the level of your Adam's apple. It may be useful to close your eyes.

Repeat this five times and check that your voice is forward in the mouth so that you can feel a slight tingle or vibration on your lips.

After practising this exercise for a period of time, you will be more aware of vocal cord vibration. And you may be able to bring this vibration to voiced sounds in your speech. The majority of people will need more extensive work, and this can be found in Appendix D.

Having the mouth in the right position

In Chapter 8 there is an explanation of how speech is produced, and this includes the contacts required to make various consonant sounds – for example, in order to make the b sound, you need to get your lips together. If you tend to use a 'starter' such as 'er', or 'ah', or 'you know', and the target word you are trying to say is 'butter', then your mouth is in the wrong position to make the b sound. 'Er', 'ah' and 'you' all start with open mouth sounds and so your lips are not together for the b in 'butter'. It is a good idea to check whether any starters that you use are preventing you from making the correct contacts for the words you are trying to say. When working on increasing fluency, it is important to ensure that your mouth is in the right position to say the sounds that you aim to say.

Soft contacts

Coupled with using the right mouth position is the use of soft contacts. This involves becoming aware of the contact required, and then aiming to keep that contact light, slow and relaxed. Make sure that the muscles of your tongue, lips and jaw remain relaxed and that you are not pushing or forcing the sound in your mouth or throat.

The moment of stammering

Prolonging or stretching out the first sound of a word is a technique that offers you a way of managing the moment of stammering, and thereby reducing the severity of your blocks. If you think your speech tends to be jerky and you are aiming for a smoother way of speaking, then you may find it helpful to stretch out, or prolong, the first sound of the word with a very light contact of the speech organs. You then say the rest of the word in the usual way and at a normal rate. Do not prolong the second or other sounds in the word unless you have a block on them.

As you prolong or stretch out the sound, focus on the movement of the speech organs in order to increase your awareness of easing through stammered or fluent sounds. Here are some guidelines:

- Say the first sound of the word with a very light contact and then move smoothly on to the next sound in the word.
- Think about keeping the tongue, lips and jaw relaxed.
- Start with words that you find easy and on which you do not expect to stammer.
- Be aware of the sounds that can be prolonged easily. This includes certain consonants and all the vowel sounds, for example – e as in every, ee (eeevening), f (fffour), i (iiin), l (llloud), m (mmmore), n (nnnine) o (ooover), r (rrrose), s (sssseven), u (uuunder) v (vvvery), w (wwwhen), y (yyyou), z (zzzoo).
- When first practising with reading, prolong approximately every fourth or fifth word – there is no hard and fast rule.

Begin with reading until you become familiar with the sounds that can be prolonged. This may feel strange at first, but you will soon find it comes quite easily. Eventually, you will be able to take this new skill to words on which you stammer. You will have more awareness of the movements of your tongue, lips and jaw so that, at this later stage, you can transfer this awareness to a stammered sound and, by releasing the tension in the speech organs, you can ease gently through the stammer and into the word.

Section 3 – Covert stammering

Self-talk or what you are thinking

Self-talk is what you say to yourself in your thoughts – like a running commentary which goes on throughout your life. When you think about it, you talk more to yourself than to anyone else!

Positive self-talk is when you tell yourself things like 'I can do it', 'I am going to try', 'I'm an OK person', 'I'm good at my job', or 'I like myself'. Conversely, negative self-talk occurs when you put yourself down with thoughts such as 'I can't do it', 'I always get it wrong', 'My presentation was terrible', 'I know I'm going to fail', 'They all thought I was stupid'.

Many people who stammer complain of a lack of confidence or of low self-esteem. If your self-talk is positive, you will give yourself confidence, self-esteem and energy; if it is negative, you can make yourself feel miserable, inadequate and incapable. This is because self-talk is accepted by your brain as being true, whereas, although it can be partly true, it is rarely, if ever, the whole truth. Take the following example:

Harry

Harry works in an open-plan office with 20-plus other employees. He reported that he always thinks that every worker is listening to his stammer when he makes a telephone call. Harry was helped to become more realistic about this situation. He discovered that most people were busy with their own work, and that the two people either side of him were aware of his stammer, but not particularly interested or bothered.

Certain self-statements become automatic over the years and you are probably unaware of what you are telling yourself. If you are worried about answering the telephone, you may not realize that you automatically think, 'The phone is ringing, I can't answer it, I feel terrible, I know there will just be a long silence'. You have had these thoughts so often when the telephone rings that you no longer consider them.

Changing the way that you think – sometimes called cognitive change – necessitates working in stages. Your aim is to change from a negative to a more realistic and positive attitude. To achieve this you will need to break up both conscious and automatic self-talk by becoming more mindful of what you are telling yourself, and asking yourself, 'Is this realistic? Reasonable?', 'Do I really have any evidence that this is true?'

The first stage is to catch these often fleeting and automatic thoughts. One way of doing this is to keep a daily record. (Record sheets and advice are given in Appendix E.)

Remind yourself that you were not born with the thoughts that you have now. These thoughts have grown and multiplied over the years as you began to worry about your stammer. They are *your* thoughts. With hard work, *you* can change them.

Reducing avoidance behaviours

All adults who stammer use avoidance strategies to varying degrees, and work on reducing such avoidance is almost always relevant. The late Professor Joseph Sheehan, who himself stammered, developed a therapy approach centred around avoidance reduction because he believed that stammering is largely maintained by the speaker's attempts *not* to stammer. Over the years, so many secondary strategies have crept into the speech of adults that it is difficult to find, or remember, the crucial core behaviour. The harder the person tries not to stammer, the more difficult speaking becomes.

Coping with reducing your avoidance behaviours requires considerable courage because it involves accepting your stammer and yourself as a person who stammers. You will need to approach some of your difficult situations instead of avoiding them, and slowly but surely reduce the fear of stammering, and the fear of being heard to stammer.

When devising your own stammering 'iceberg' and 'onion', you will have discovered the extent of your own secondary behaviours – and perhaps have also become aware of how many tricks and tactics you use to hide your stammer. You use these because you have always considered episodes of fluent speech to be a success, regardless of how that fluency was achieved, and instances of stammering to be a failure. We are now suggesting that you rethink this mental set by teaching yourself to accept your stammer rather than hiding and avoiding it. In the long term, this will give you freedom and peace of mind.

Give some time and thought to Sheehan's list of avoidance reduction concepts:

- Your stammering is a conflict between going ahead and holding back.
- To improve, you must reduce, and finally get rid of, the holding back.

- To improve, you must reduce, and finally get rid of, your habits of avoidance and hiding.
- Your stammering is a 'false-role' disorder. You will remain a stammerer as long as you continue to pretend not to be one.
- You have a choice as to *how* you stammer. You may not always have a choice as to *when* you stammer.
- You can choose to stammer openly and smoothly.
- What you call your 'stammer' consists mostly of the tricks and crutches you use to cover up.
- Your stammer is like an iceberg – much of the difficulty is kept concealed below the surface, inside yourself. If you get more of it above the surface, you will get rid of it more easily.
- Reducing your tricks of avoidance is not a process you need to keep working on for ever. You have learnt or acquired a set of attitudes, feelings and habits; you can learn a new set.

Avoidances

1 Ask yourself whether avoidances have helped you in the long run or just got you out of a difficult situation for that moment?

2 Make sure you have identified, and are clear about, the secondary behaviours that constitute your avoidances.

3 Make a list of what you do, or refer to your list in Chapter 7.

4 Score every successful task that you complete in open stammering.

5 Choose one of the following to work on – always start with whatever is easiest for you:

- Twice a day, establish eye contact before speaking.
- Once a day, keep eye contact while stammering.
- Deliberately use one feared word per day instead of changing that word to something you can say without stammering.
- Complete three feared words per day.
- Three times a day, count silently to three before starting to speak.
- Talk to one person about your stammer.
- Pick one feared speaking situation and do it in spite of your fear.

You can find more exercises in Appendix F.

You can now continue to choose other ideas in the above list and set your own targets as to how many words or situations per day or per week you will do. You can be very proud of yourself for doing this work, so stay with it and be patient – we promise that it will be well worthwhile.

- The more you run away from your stammering, the more you will stammer. The more you are open and courageous, the more you will develop solid fluency.
- In accepting yourself as a stammerer you choose the route to becoming a more honest and relaxed speaker.

How many of these concepts do you agree with? Why? Which do you disagree with? Why?

If you want to try open stammering, there is no time like the present. Be sure to work step by step – you have relied on avoidance for a long time and the reduction of this behaviour must be done slowly and gently.

How to reduce avoidances? This is not an easy thing to do, but – in the future – you will be delighted to find that the actions you now take will be with you for life.

Some suggestions are given in the box on page 80.

Finally ... the secret of success

Regardless of the work you have chosen to do, what would you say is the secret for success? We think that it is to practise, practise and practise, and not give up. This can seem a very facile piece of advice when you may feel that others can just talk when and how they want, while you have to go through all of this. For better or worse, that is the reality for you. In order to speak with ease at those meetings, for your presentation, during an exam or with a special friend, you will need to think about what you are doing and practise in the easy situations on your hierarchy. And then practise some more as you progress up your ladder towards the more difficult situations. The secret of success is not magic or anything special, it is what you would do in any other sphere of life – practise. After all, you do not expect to play in a tennis tournament, at a concert, sit for an exam or run the marathon without practising. Consistent, motivated practice will help you to reach whatever goal you are aiming to achieve.

Main points in this chapter

- Increasing fluency.
- Breathing.
- Vocal cord or vocal fold work.
- Correct mouth position.
- Soft contacts.
- The moment of stammering.
- Self-talk.
- Reducing avoidance.

12

Additional sources of help

If you live in the UK, a wide range of resources may be available to you, and it can be confusing to decide which of these would be the most helpful. This chapter aims to provide brief information on some of the options, and we must stress that space does not allow for mention of all possible sources.

All the contact details for organizations, individuals and websites mentioned in this chapter can be found in the Useful addresses section, and there are recommended books in the Further reading list to accompany some of the topics mentioned. The British Stammering Association (BSA) website offers independent information on most items, either directly or through suggested links at <www.stammering.org> .

Speech and language therapy (SLT)

The SLT techniques that we have described previously in this book should be available free in the UK on the NHS. However, there are long waiting lists in some areas of the country and a number of authorities currently do not provide any service to adults who stammer. It is preferable to receive therapy from a SLT who specializes in stammering, and the BSA holds a list of such SLTs working in the NHS and privately.

If you choose to see a SLT privately the cost of assessment is in the region of £85 to £120 per session and on-going therapy around £40 to £70 per hour. The therapist will advise you of the fees. In order to locate a private therapist in your area, you can contact your local SLT department or the Association of Speech and Language Therapists in Independent Practice.

Most therapists offer therapy individually, but some also provide group work on a once-a-week basis, or intensively every day for one or two weeks. The advantages of being in a group can include opportunities to meet others who stammer, and the chance to practise therapy techniques in an understanding atmosphere before transferring them to the outside world. Groups can also be a great deal more fun and, whatever the technique, they are an ideal way to gain mutual support and encouragement, and to reduce feelings of isolation.

Speech and language therapists in the UK are registered by the Health Professions Council (HPC) and, in the rare event that you have a complaint about your treatment, you can contact the SLT's employer or the HPC who will investigate your concerns.

National specialist centres

The City Literary Institute (City Lit) is an adult education centre which has a SLT department that is a national specialist centre for the treatment of adults who stammer. The City Lit provides assessment, evening classes and intensive courses and, although not residential, its facilities are available to anyone living outside the area as well as for Londoners. You can contact the City Lit directly or through your SLT.

<www.citylit.ac.uk/stammeringtherapy>

The Michael Palin Centre for Stammering Children (MPC) is also a national specialist centre which gives a comprehensive service, including intensive courses. The MPC can be accessed through the NHS and referrals are accepted from any part of the UK for children, young people up to the age of 19, and parents.

<www.stammeringcentre.org>

Non-professional courses

There are some intensive group courses available for adults that are not run by SLTs, but frequently by people who themselves stammered and now wish to help others. These courses charge fees of between £250 and £700, excluding hotel accommodation.

We have described throughout this book how stammering is highly individual in nature and that the most effective therapy is designed to meet your specific needs. Commercial courses tend to provide a one-size-fits-all approach and do not generally undertake individual assessment before enrolling people on their courses. Therefore, you are advised to find out as much as you can about the treatment methods, long-term support, and whether the approach would suit your type of stammer.

The best known of these courses are perhaps the following:

The McGuire Programme. This was devised by David McGuire who himself stammered, and is now run by people who stammer and for people who stammer. McGuire himself comes from a sports background, and basic to the programme is the principle that participants are athletes training to become proficient at their 'sport' – the sport of speaking.

This programme aims to promote self-acceptance and effective communication skills, and combines a number of techniques. Central is a specific form of breathing coupled with the necessity to continue 'training' or practising for as long as it is necessary to change previous speaking patterns and gain speech control.

Four-day, intensive, residential courses are held in large groups throughout the UK and in other parts of the world. After the initial course, candidates become lifelong members of the organization and follow-up attendance is an integral part of the programme.

<www.mcguireprogramme.com>

The Starfish Project. This was founded by Anne Blight when she moved away from working on the McGuire programme. The principle of her approach is to use a technique, based on a specific breathing pattern, in order to replace stammering with controlled speech and with the management of negative feelings that have developed around the stammer. The aim is to provide candidates with a 'toolbox' of approaches so that a variety of methods are available to use in different speaking situations.

This programme is offered as a three-day intensive, residential course and is held in small groups so that individual attention is a feature. On-going help is accessible by means of a further free-of-charge course, telephone contact with someone trained in the technique, or a support group formed to continue work on the Starfish approach.

<www.starfishproject.co.uk>

Self-help groups

Some stammerers gain great support from attending a self-help group during, following or instead of therapy. Such a group can provide opportunities to meet others who stammer and access mutual support and encouragement.

Self-help groups vary in size, structure and activities. The BSA can provide information about available groups or, if you are considering starting one up yourself, they will provide a pack on how to do this, as well as guidelines on how to run it successfully.

If you are unable to access a group near where you live, or find the prospect of entering a group too daunting, you can contact, via email, others who stammer. The BSA provides information on ways of making contact for friendship and support via the self-help pages of their website, or you can email them:

<e-friends@stammering.org>

Speaking Circles

Speaking Circles were devised to help anyone who is uncomfortable speaking in a group, regardless of whether that group is a tutorial, presentation, meeting or any other gathering. The technique used in Speaking Circles is simple and straightforward. It is mainly based on giving support and full attention to the speaker, as opposed to criticism, lack of attention or judgemental advice – such advice has been the unfortunate experience of many who are afraid of public speaking.

This method proved so successful that people who stammered became involved and found the system extremely useful because it allows space to develop your own way of speaking in public, allows you to be yourself, and increases confidence.

The key principles of Speaking Circles are:

- learning to slow down and listen attentively both to yourself and your audience;
- starting to trust in yourself, and in the fact that what you have to say is valuable;
- making a connection with your audience;
- increasing your ability to make that connection with the audience;
- discovering how to tolerate silence and pauses.

<www.speakingcircles.com>

Speakers Clubs and Toastmasters

These are two further organizations that are not aimed specifically at stammering, but exist to help people in general improve their skills and confidence in public speaking and giving presentations. You can join a local group, as an observer initially, then ultimately make short speeches, progressing at your own pace. Fellow members offer support and constructive feedback. Many people who stammer have found this to be a helpful way to practise public speaking and you can find a local group via their respective websites in Useful addresses.

<www.toastmasters.org>

<www.the-asc.org.uk>

Social skills and assertiveness training

We have mentioned in previous chapters the fact that effective communication is not dependent upon fluent speech. Improving your social skills can help you to communicate more effectively – perhaps to a level that is better than your fluent colleagues and friends, regardless of your stammer. This can be helpful both socially and at work.

Attending a course or reading a book on how to improve social skills may address such areas as:

- Personal distance and posture
- Eye contact, facial expression and gesture
- Loudness and tone of voice
- Rate and use of pausing
- Improving listening skills
- How to start and end conversations
- Keeping conversations going
- Making friends
- Job interviews and giving presentations.

Assertive behaviour is a social skill, and learning to behave more assertively can be particularly helpful for people lacking in confidence and self-esteem. Being assertive can be misunderstood as being aggressive, but assertiveness training can help to differentiate between aggressive and assertive behaviours. Assertive behaviour will enable you to:

- express your ideas and feelings, both positive and negative, in an open, direct and honest manner;
- stand up for your rights while respecting the rights of others;
- take responsibility for yourself and your actions without judging or blaming others;
- find a compromise where conflict exists.

All the above may be skills that you have not had a chance to develop previously due to your stammer – enhancing them may not only make you a more effective communicator, but also increase your general self-confidence.

There are many self-help books available on the subject, but you may find it useful to enrol on a course as it helps to practise the skills required in a supportive environment before trying them out in the real world. See Further reading for some suggested self-help books.

Relaxation

Most people who stammer experience some tension in the muscles of the face and neck while stammering, and many find that the tension spreads to other parts of the body. If a person stammers very severely and continuously, they may have forgotten what it feels like to have muscles that are relaxed and at ease. Being continually tense is exhausting, and physical tension often goes hand in hand with anxiety and mental tension.

Relaxation or meditation work is not just helpful for your stammer – a calmer mind and body will enhance other areas of your life. It can help to relieve stress, manage anxiety, restore energy levels and promote health. Not everyone is either interested or suited to this work, but it is worth giving this aspect some consideration.

There are many forms of mental and physical relaxation on offer and there is a large range of information available on the internet, in books, on CDs and DVDs, as well as at classes. Most methods fall into two broad categories: physical and psychological approaches. If you are someone who can easily close your eyes and conjure up a relaxing image that helps to calm you down, you may prefer a mental approach. If, on the other hand, you prefer bodily activity as a way to let off steam, you may find a physical approach suits you best.

You will probably be aware of some of the methods currently available – yoga, reiki, reflexology, tai-chi, Pilates, massage, a workout in the gym and others too numerous to name. All of these have been found of help to some. You may need to experiment with a variety of techniques until you discover what suits you best.

Certain SLTs teach general relaxation, and learning how to relax the muscles used in speech can be one aspect of speech modification techniques. Some of the approaches mentioned need to be taught by a skilled practitioner, while others can be learnt from audio, video, CDs or DVD recordings. Whichever approach you try, you are advised to practise regularly so as to gain sufficient expertise to transfer the benefits to your everyday life. Relaxation is not a quick fix, but a strategy that can have many widespread benefits.

You may find it useful to do a quick check of the trigger points for tension:

Tongue Gravity dictates that when the tongue is relaxed, it will rest on the floor of the mouth. The tongue is a muscle, and if you find that it is held in the roof of your mouth then there is tension. Release the tension and let the tongue fall down to the floor of the mouth.

Shoulders   If you are hunched up or the shoulders are rather nearer to your ears than they should be, release the tension. Shrug the shoulders up towards your ears and then let them drop. Do that two or three times.

Hands   Are they clenched or gripped tightly together? Let them fall loosely by your side or on to your lap.

Legs   Are you one of those people who push their legs into the floor? Do you tap your feet? Tense the calf muscles? If so, release that tension and let the floor take the weight of your feet.

You could make a start by noting those trigger points at various times during your day, especially when in a traffic jam, waiting in a queue or facing a difficult situation.

Meditation

Meditation is closely related to relaxation, but perhaps more concerned with calming the mind than the muscles of the body. Mind and body are closely linked, so that you cannot have tense muscles and a relaxed mind – nor vice versa. It is virtually impossible for us to think of nothing and to just blank our minds; therefore, most meditative practices centre on focusing our attention on one thing – a flickering candle, special music, a colour, a mantra or our breathing.

The two forms of meditation that are well known in the UK at this time are:

1 *Mindfulness*. Meditation is about being awake to, and aware of, thoughts, feelings and sensations as they occur right here and now. We often live in the past and think about events that have been and gone, or in the future by predicting what could happen about something that is yet to occur. We may forget that the only time we actually experience life is in each moment as it unfolds. If our minds are always miles away rather than in the present moment, we can miss any number of interesting happenings, and we can become tense and stressed worrying about the past and the future, while missing the present.

   Mindfulness is practised daily either sitting, lying, standing or moving, and is developed by deliberately paying attention to what is happening at the present moment. A central quality of this work is being non-judgemental and accepting the present because it is here. Practitioners of this method find that they learn to look at life in a different way and achieve a calmness, patience and acceptance that they had not previously experienced.

<www.mindfulness-meditation.net>

2   *Transcendental Meditation (TM)*. This is a unique technique that has been practised by millions of people throughout the world since its foundation in 1957. It is a technique that is both simple to learn and to practise, and it is taught in an identical, systematic manner throughout the world. It is advisable to practise for 20 minutes twice a day and, as you are sitting in silence, it is quite possible to do this on a train or bus journey. TM offers long-term benefits by giving deep rest to mind and body through the use of a natural way of releasing tiredness and stress.

Among a number of reported benefits, people practising this method say that their physical and mental energy is increased, their stress levels are reduced, and their effectiveness in everyday situations is enhanced. There are classes available in most areas of the UK and in other parts of the world, as well as books for teaching this approach.

<www.t-m.org.uk>

Hypnosis

It may be surprising to some to realize that we often experience trance states during the course of our lives – passing into ordinary sleep involves a kind of trance state. The experience of hypnosis is similar: neither asleep nor awake and a little like daydreaming, with a pleasant feeling of deep relaxation behind it all. Hypnosis is a different state of consciousness into which you can enter naturally so that, for therapeutic purposes (hypnotherapy), valuable suggestions may be given directly to your unconscious mind. People can also be taught self-hypnosis and, for some, this can be an effective means of relaxation.

The idea of alleviating stammering through hypnosis is extremely attractive but, unfortunately, the success rate does not seem high. There are difficulties in assessing the contribution of hypnosis because hypnotists who have worked with people who stammer and claimed their treatment was successful do not give adequate information.

Regrettably there is also almost no legislation in the UK designed to regulate the training and qualification of hypnotherapy practitioners. The quality of training varies enormously, and the organizations listed in Useful addresses provide advice on finding a practitioner who has a high standard of training, undergoes supervision, and abides by a code of ethics with a formal complaints procedure.

<www.bsch.org.uk>

<www.nrhp.co.uk>

Counselling

Counselling is a form of talking therapy that allows individuals the chance to converse about the problems in their lives, and discuss difficult feelings, relationships and situations with a qualified listener in a safe and confidential environment. Most people benefit from talking therapies because they can do for the mind what exercise does for the body – increase your energy, help you to think with greater clarity, make you stronger emotionally, and prevent more serious problems from occurring.

The word 'counselling' covers a wide range of therapies and these may be offered in depth by a highly trained counsellor, or by an SLT on a more basic level as part of the treatment for stammering. Every year many people seek counselling as it becomes more and more acceptable to obtain professional help for personal concerns.

It can be difficult to find your way to the kind of counsellor who will be best able to help you, but it is important to make an informed choice about the options available and, in order to do this, you will require information. Such detailed information is outside the range of this book, but we would advise investigating the situation by doing one or more of the following: consulting your GP, your SLT, the British Association for Counselling and Psychotherapy (BACP), Citizens Advice Bureau, obtaining a personal recommendation, or reading a book (see Further reading).

As with all aspects of stammering, some people have been helped greatly by counselling, others not at all. Finding the right type of counselling, and a counsellor to suit your needs, may be an important factor in ensuring success.

<www.bacp.co.uk>

Neuro-Linguistic Programming (NLP)

The name 'Neuro-Linguistic Programming' is somewhat of a mouthful, but the approach is clear and logical, and some find it effective. The name was originally chosen to describe the technique because:

Neuro – refers to how the mind and body interact.

Linguistic – describes how careful listening to the way that language is used can give us insight into the way another person is thinking.

Programming – expresses the patterns and habitual behaviours that people use to organize their everyday lives.

Although NLP is simple on one level, it is quite complex on another, so it is best to attend a course or classes where you can learn the method fully. If that is impossible for you, there are informative books that will be useful and lead you through a series of exercises to acquire the skills of this approach.

A basic principle of this method is the study of factors that account for either success and achievement or failure and disappointment and, through this study, various ways of thinking and behaving have been established that help everyone, fluent or stammering, to be more successful and effective in all areas of their lives.

<mike.reprogram@connectfree.co.uk>

Medication/drug treatment

There is currently no medication available in the UK that can be prescribed specifically to help reduce stammering, although some doctors have prescribed tranquillizers or beta-blockers to help people cope with anxiety related to their stammering. This type of medication may prove helpful in combination with other therapy approaches, but any side effects or long-term consequences need to be considered.

Studies are on-going in the USA with a drug called pagoclone, which has not yet been made commercially available. This drug improved fluency in some and had an anxiety-reducing effect, but there are side effects such as headache and fatigue. Researchers in this area feel that future treatment will probably involve the combination of medication with speech and language therapy to achieve the optimal results.

Drug therapy for stammering is in its infancy, and treatment through medication is still remote. There have been no large-scale controlled research studies of any drug therapies, and even if they were completed successfully, current licensing arrangements would take several years before prescription could be available in the UK.

Electronic devices and software

Some people who stammer find that they can speak fluently when reading or speaking in unison with another person, or if they cannot hear their voices due to background noise. There are electronic devices on the market that imitate this effect with the help of earphones, which alter the pitch of the voice or relay the voice back to the speaker with a fraction of a second's delay. The combined effect is to make it sound as if you have a voice speaking in your ear while talking. Alternatively, some devices mask the sound of the voice with a hiss or a buzz.

The only way to discover whether one of these devices will affect your fluency is to try one. Some people find that the effect is immediate, others take longer to learn to concentrate on the sound and let it guide their speech. For some, the devices have no effect on their speech at all.

These appliances vary in size and design. Some are small in-ear devices which look like a tiny hearing aid, while others are the size of an iPod and are used with a microphone and earpiece like a hands-free set for a mobile phone. The cost ranges from around £200 to over £3,000, depending on their sizes and what they offer. A few can be purchased on a trial basis, but others recommend that they are fitted by a SLT who is trained in how to fine-tune the device and provide help and support.

When considering whether you would like to try one of these appliances it may be helpful to consider the following questions:

- Will you be comfortable being seen wearing it?
- Will you be able to cope with a continuous sound in your ear like a voice or a buzz?
- How effectively will the device work on the telephone, in noisy environments, or if you are anxious?
- Will the device be activated if you block silently and do not produce voice when you stammer?

Independent research is being carried out on the long-term effectiveness of such devices. In general, the advice is that none of them should be seen as a cure, but rather as an added tool because they appear to be most effective when used in conjunction with other therapy techniques.

More information about the devices available can be obtained via the BSA website:

<www.stammering.org/adther_electronicaids.html>

This website also includes information on various software packages available for installation on desktop computers, handheld computers and mobile phones that provide altered auditory feedback.

For those interested in using software as a therapy programme, there is a computerized fluency-shaping programme called Dr Fluency, which aims to provide home-based training for slow prolonged speech.

<www.drfluency.com>

Disability Discrimination Act

In the UK, stammering is sometimes covered by the Disability Discrimination Act (1995), so if you feel that you have experienced discrimination, you may find the following website helpful:

<www.stammeringlaw.org.uk>

Main points in this chapter

- Sources of speech and language therapy.
- Non-professional courses.
- Self-help and email groups.
- Speaking Circles.
- Speakers Clubs and Toastmasters.
- Relaxation and meditation.
- Social skills and assertiveness training.
- Hypnosis.
- Counselling.
- Neuro-Linguistic Programming (NLP).
- Medication/drug treatment.
- Electronic devices and software.
- Disability Discrimination Act.

13

From those who stammer

Iona – age five (written by her mother)

Iona was born in 2002 and for her first two years she showed no interest in trying to speak, was happy with her own company, and hated visiting new places. She wasn't frustrated, and just let her sister say everything for her. At the age of two we had our first visit to our local speech and language therapist. She spent a good two hours with Iona and us and was a calming influence, giving us lots of advice and handy tips. We started Iona early in a pre-school to encourage communication without us around, and dance and swimming clubs to build confidence. The next year was spent with regular visits to our therapist and, by her third birthday, Iona was finally saying a single word, singing and making animal sounds. We began to use Makaton signing, which was great for all the family to learn and Iona loved it.

Gradually, Iona progressed to two words together – she was relaxed and uninterested until we made words funny. Finally, when asked what does Aunty Judy have? She would reply 'big bum' – a huge breakthrough, and more words came, but then we hit another problem – Iona began to stammer! It was a constant worry that there was something wrong in her brain, but our therapist did continual small tests with Iona to ascertain her understanding and these showed there were no problems.

Our speech and language therapist was brilliant and gave us huge encouragement, but Iona's stammering got worse and we were asked to plot a daily graph to see if there was any pattern in her good and bad days. It was hard work to allow Iona time to get her words out and at times she would get upset, get halfway through saying some words, and just give up and then say clearly 'Oh, it doesn't matter' without a single stammer! Slowly a pattern started to show from our daily graph – any form of excitement made the stammering worse, particularly Christmas and her birthday.

At the beginning we ignored the stammering so as not to draw attention to it, but when Iona got upset about it the therapist started to call them 'bumpy words' and 'smooth words' and encouraged her that it didn't matter. We were also shown how to slow Iona down and get her to concentrate on what she wanted to say. By the age of three and a half, Iona had good and bad days, but even the good days would still have some stammering. We began to believe Iona would stammer for life. Then, when she was about four, the stammering got less and less and, when we got to the excitement of Christmas, she did not stammer but just repeated some words. After Christmas 2006 it just disappeared and has never come back. Our therapist believes the stammering began because Iona was late to talk and finally developed with her words too fast, and then couldn't say them quickly enough.

It was a huge concern for us and there were times I thought she would never be able to read a book at school, and yet now she is so outgoing and is reading beautifully. All this was down to an excellent speech and language therapist with the right ideas.

Tom – age 11

The disadvantage of having a stammer is that if you are still at school, you could get bullied or teased about it. You just need to shake it off because there is nothing wrong with you – it is just your speech. You may get frustrated if your stammer is bad and you might get stuck sometimes, but there are strategies to help you keep smooth – and in some ways they might make you feel like you don't have a stammer at all.

Tom's mother

Tom has been living with a stammer for six years, although it is fair to say that as a family we all live with his stammer. Tom has therapy when he feels the need but, mostly, he is comfortable just as he is. This hasn't always been the case, and over the years Tom has been victimized and bullied for 'being different'. If I could have kept him home and wrapped in cotton wool during these difficult periods, then that's exactly what I would have done.

Tom went on an intensive speech and language therapy course where we met with other families. We both enjoyed the freedom that comes with being around other people who understand – it's a shame there isn't a support group in our area. It's been a difficult road, with bullying hidden round the odd corner and clouds of low self-esteem overhead, but for the most part Tom is comfortable walking in his own shoes. I couldn't be more proud of my son!

Matt – age 16

My name is Matt and I am 16 years old. At a first glance people may think of me as any old average Joe walking down the street. On many occasions I find these early assumptions cruelly replaced whenever I have to talk to people for the first time. People often get confused, annoyed, embarrassed and impatient – or simply laugh at me when I have to respond to a question that my mouth just won't allow me to answer.

For me, stammering has always been a major problem in my life. It has previously stopped me from doing simple things that other people take for granted, such as talking on the telephone, answering a question in class, meeting new people, or asking for assistance in a shop. From the outside, many people who I know come to a conclusion that my stammer isn't that big a problem – but for me it is. If you could look inside my mind you would find there are a lot of emotional problems for me that go with having a stammer. From about the age six I can remember worrying about my stammer and what people thought of me. I would often get very depressed and feel very alone. I had never met another person with the same problem. Stammering is a very complex thing to have to deal with. Sometimes I can go for days and even weeks where I can speak completely fluently and only stammering a few times a day, and other days can be really bad and I can hardly say a word. When I have bad days I always get very uptight and frustrated with myself, which can make me depressed for days at a time. The main problem concerning my stammer that makes me very angry is when I want to say something really important or ask a question in class, and the thought of stammering makes me avoid the situation, which makes me feel really low.

I knew I couldn't let stammering affect me for the whole of my life and I had come to accept the fact that it was never going to go away and was always going to be a part of who I am. But I knew that there were fluency techniques and strategies you can learn, which put you in control of the stammer rather than the stammer being in control of you. The ones that particularly worked miracles for me were techniques called slow speech and soft contacts.

Luckily for me my speech and language therapist was able to arrange for me to take part in a two-week intensive course. This course really helped me to become in control of my stammer. I gained a whole load of confidence from the experience from the course. But the main thing I learnt, which has perhaps changed my life for ever, is that I am not alone – there are other people out there going through the same difficulties as me. If I could give a message to others that suffer from a stammer, it would be: as long as you remain positive and remember that you aren't alone, there is no reason why you can't achieve all you want to achieve in life. Never let stammering get in the way of your dreams and what you want to do in life.

Felicity – age 23

I feel intensely negative towards my stammer. To the outside world I appear fluent, happy and confident; inside I am constantly carrying around the burden of ensuring that as few people as possible find out about the stammer I've been hiding for as long as I can remember. There have been so many times in life where I have avoided situations that would involve me having to speak to people I do not know. I will always remember one incident at university when my wallet went missing and I refused to phone up and cancel my cards. The thought of having to phone up my card company and tell them my details over the phone was more frightening to me than the idea someone could have access to my bank account.

I have learnt over the years to control my stammer in normal conversation to the point where I speak fluently – until, that is, someone asks me to say my name, or I have to make a phone call. Then I feel all the anxiety symptoms creeping up and my stammer takes over. I am quite often paralysed with fear when I hear my mobile phone ringing and I refuse to pick it up for days. For me, what is most distressing is that I would love nothing more than to be able to take up acting for a career. However, I find that it is when I am unable to use the avoidance techniques that I have perfected for so many years in normal conversation that the true extent of my problem comes out. Therefore when I attempt to read from a script I tend to find myself in real difficulties. I have just completed a Masters degree which involved a great deal of acting at drama school and I found it the most excruciatingly painful year of my life as I struggled every week trying to act from words that were put in front of me. Yes, I had negative comments. Yes, I put myself under a huge amount of stress. I survived, but it has taken me a great deal of time to realize just how brave I was to do that.

I do believe in a strange way that stammering is a gift. I am so much more aware of other people and their feelings because of my heightened awareness of myself. When I have done something that involves me speaking out, I get a huge sense of satisfaction – greater, I am sure, than that any fluent speaker would have doing the same task. Having said that, I do find stammering incredibly difficult to live with, and more so as I have grown older. I continue to be resentful of it to a great degree, and of myself for not being able to control it to the extent that I would wish. But I will get there one day. We all will! And I truly believe that.

Cliff – age 28

Like me, many people may not have gone for help because they thought that their stammer was too mild and that the NHS would have nothing to offer. Although my stammer would be considered very mild and probably not noticed by most people, it has been a constant worry to me because I never know when it is going to hit me, which usually happens at the most inconvenient moments – like when I want to impress my bosses or a girlfriend, or when I'm in a hurry and need to say something quickly. I have never been able to rely on my speech doing the right thing.

Two years ago a friend told me about some evening classes for stammerers and, after much hesitation, I got in touch. That's one of the best things I ever did because I went to those classes every week for nearly a year and met lots of people in the same boat as myself. The therapist was great and I learnt all about interiorized stammering, which is what I have got, and learnt about how to be much more open about it rather than hiding and worrying all the time. I'm still in touch with quite a few people from that group and we meet occasionally and give each other a bit of support. It's odd because, although I do still occasionally stammer, it never worries me any more because I know what to do about it. Don't hesitate – go and get some help – it's worth it.

Robert – age 38

Having a stammer is hard, very hard – at times, indescribably hard. I have had a stammer all my life. There are many reasons for having a stammer, but it doesn't matter why you have one, what does matter is that you don't let it affect your life. If you want to speak more fluently and easily, it will not happen by itself; you need to do something about it.

In my case, I found a great speech and language therapist who had the patience to spend several years with a client who was busy at work, getting married and raising a family. Gradually, we hit the stammer from the emotional and the technical angles. By far the most difficult was the emotional dimension. I had built up so much tension, worries and fears over the years, and these had to be encountered and talked through before I could really hit the stammer.

I have gone from being an aspiring lawyer who was told not to practise law because of the stammer, to being a leading lawyer in an internet company. Your stammer need not define you; you and your intelligence and skills are so much more than your stammer. So, I implore you to do whatever you really want to do and never avoid anything because of your stammer. Do I still get nervous before speaking in public? You bet I do, but here's the point – so do most people. Do I speak completely fluently? No. But will I talk confidently, look people in the eye, and be more than my stammer? Yes, I bloody well will!

I try and remember three things, but I don't always succeed:

1 Never try and be fluent, just try and speak easily and without tension.
2 Pause, always pause. It's so tempting to rush and finish off what you're saying and not stammer. If you rush, and don't take your time, you will run out of breath and stammer. I do.
3 Don't allow tension to creep into your speech because that's what it does. Unless you're watching for it, it creeps back. Try not to widen your mouth too much and don't talk too loudly, just speak gently.

Everyone is different, and everyone will have their two or three main things to watch for. You will have yours and, if you want to, use them and speak more fluently and easily. And if you still stammer, it doesn't matter, you're still great and, by the way, much better than that other bloke or woman who talks crap in a boring grey, monotone which bores everyone to sleep!

One more thing. My daughter developed a stammer at the age of three and a half. It was my worst fear come to life. We were made aware of an amazing programme aimed at children, called the Lidcombe Program. Within six months of very light-touch speech and language therapy and practice time, my daughter's stammer had completely gone and now, four years later, she speaks beautifully and confidently. It can be done.

Jonathan – age 38

I have stammered since the age of six. I still stammer today, but my relationship with my stammer is one of understanding and respect. My stammer is part of my character.

My early memories were of acute embarrassment, with an inability to say my name or answer the register. I learnt techniques to avoid speaking or to force words out by brute force. I can remember the physical exhaustion of any kind of public speaking.

At the age of six, I saw a speech and language therapist, but did not like the technique she taught me and, aged 12, I went to see a hypnotherapist, but that did not help either.

Throughout this time fear gripped my every public moment and I felt alone and depressed. Then things improved and I gained acceptance with my peers; and although I still stammered, it became less of an obstacle and I spent less time in self-pity. Arriving at college my stammer flared up again – stammers are like that! Fellow students thought I was putting it on for a laugh. One student who became a good friend recognized what was going on and said it was one of the bravest things he had ever seen. That made me feel good.

Going out to work meant that I had to use the phone and interviews are also part of the process. Tension was at the fore and I was unable to express myself, and I left interviews feeling physically drained. Jobs did come – and, again, an initial period of stammering was followed by more fluent speech. While at college I had discovered that alcohol seemed to cure both my nerves and stammer.

Gradually, my stammer improved to the outside world. I used advanced techniques for avoiding sounds and places. My family commented on how my speech had improved. There were still those moments, though, when out of the blue I would block and stammer.

When I was 28 I decided to give speech and language therapy a go. I just wanted to dive in. However, I needed to be assessed and I spent an uncomfortable hour with a speech and language therapist. This led to an evening course, but listening to others stammering was so shameful – I'm embarrassed by that statement now – how full of pride I was.

At 32 my stammer returned. I was beaten and decided to take two weeks out and attend an intensive course of speech and language therapy. My employer was supportive. On this course I was desensitized, taught how to form sounds correctly, was encouraged to stammer openly and not to hide away. It was scary being videoed – lack of eye contact, blocking, face pulling and repetition. But I did it, and by the end of the two weeks I had acceptance that I stammered and felt good. I also had a whole set of exercises and tools to use.

Today I use those tools. I almost enjoy reading aloud and I keep in touch with other stammerers. I still stammer (not much), but I speak when I like. The key was giving in to my stammer and seeking help.

Lucy – age 39

I have no recollection of not stammering, although my parents say that it started around the age of four or five. I was the youngest in a very competitive family, and my brothers, who are very strong characters, took very much centre stage and much of my parents' time. I remember being desperate to be able to talk and being talked over, so I feel that I developed my stammer probably as a nervous reaction to being constantly interrupted and not listened to all the way through. I must admit that I wasn't very concerned about my stammer when I was very young – I had many friends and didn't feel at all self-conscious about it. My parents, however, were obviously concerned and took me to see many different speech and language therapists, all offering something different and their own advice and methods of conquering the speech impediment. I think that this probably made me switch off completely to speech therapy at a young age and I continued almost to rebel against any sort of help with my speech for the whole of my young life until my early thirties.

I had a very good school life (I went to boarding school at the age of 11) and my only real frustration was not feeling able to audition for school musicals, especially as I had a very good singing voice, but the speaking part always felt like a huge barrier for me. I then went on to have a year in the States working for the White House administration, and then returned to work for ten years in the City of London. Both companies I worked for are extremely fast moving and one of my roles was as a marketing co-ordinator whereby I organized conferences and road shows across Europe, travelling extensively, and regularly greeting up to 300 people a day.

I then got married and we relocated to the coast to start a family. I developed vocal nodules through my singing and was sent to a speech and language therapist to try to eradicate them without the need for surgery. Towards the end of my treatment, she asked whether my stammer ever bothered me – I replied very quickly that it didn't, but on returning home I reflected on this question and felt that I was rather kidding myself! On my next visit I mentioned that I had thought about her question and she went on to recommend a colleague who specialized in stammering, who was living nearby. I somewhat tentatively went to see her and have never looked back – it was the very best thing I have ever done and now, whenever I go through a difficult or stressful time, I now control the stammer rather than the other way round.

Marc – age 41

I have had a stammer since I was approximately seven years old. The stammer was most noticeable in secondary school in Liverpool and I believe it is linked to the death of my mother. These were very difficult years and the teachers were unable to assist.

One positive thing came out of this. I was very good at language, and found that in a second language my stammer was considerably reduced – I could also read much quicker than the other pupils, and this is still true. Over the years I have been to a number of speech and language therapists and found them helpful in understanding the complexity of the stammer. I found speaking to people about the stammer, whether family or colleagues, helped a bit, but I was conscious that I did not want to be thought of as disadvantaged.

I am now comfortable with my stammer. I manage an IT department within a banking environment and deal with conference calls and project planning. Has it stopped me in my life from achieving professional goals? Yes, probably, but I think it is important to look at the positives of what you have achieved instead of the negatives. Sometimes too much detail can make it worse, which I believe is part of the problem.

Alex – age 42

So there I am lying on the cold floor with my eyes closed and the smell of the dusty office lingering. The therapist spoke in soft tones '... and now relaxing deeper and deeper'. My mind was on one thing only – 'three pence please'.

I was 12 years of age and attending speech and language therapy. It was bad enough being the only boy with a stammer in a school full of nut-cases, but I had to leave class every week, which made me more conspicuous. But it was the fear of having to ask the bus-conductor for the fare 'three pence please' that preoccupied me most of the time. So what was I worried about – my therapist was teaching me how to relax! I thought it was strange that she never asked me how I felt, why I thought I stammered, or what was really going on ... but why would she, I was only 12 years old, what would I know?

Probably my first real therapy as an adult was in an intensive group session for six days with a hypnotist. A peculiar choice you might think, but in the early eighties choices were somewhat limited. It was probably a form of brainwashing but it helped me to see there were options, even if that one didn't work for long. Also, I got to spend a week with other stammerers and learn a lot from them. Next I attended a weekly group with student speech and language therapists at the university. Here I learnt about real techniques and was introduced to the work of Van Riper, gaining a deeper understanding of the problem.

A few years later I was in desperation, my work had me under pressure to communicate, and my job required a lot of telephone calls. I went back to the university to look at options and was directed to an intensive speech and language therapy course called 'Coping with Stammering'. This changed my life; it was here that I really understood how my feelings, beliefs and actions were linked. I learnt real techniques and coping strategies and left that course a changed person. My stammer persisted, but was mostly controlled and predictable. I learnt how to stammer openly and left the fear behind. That time on that course is treasured to this day, as it was a turning point for me in the total acceptance of my stammer.

My most recent adventure has been with narrative therapy. Here I learnt to understand the stammer as a separate 'character', and through writing I developed his character and learnt that I can actually have a life without a stammer. One thing I have learnt is that every stammerer is different and his or her needs have to be carefully identified. Also, the stammerer needs the right therapies, but only at the right time. Thirty years ago I knew a little bit, but I know a lot more now. Maybe if I had had the right help at the time, I might not have had to battle my way through so many of the following years. Now I don't worry too much about paying the bus-fare, let them wait if they have to!

Charles – age 43

My stammer isn't my enemy any more. Now we're almost friends. I've stammered all of my speaking life. I've heard a tape of me aged three and I was stammering then. I stammer overtly. I do everything – I block, I back-track, I use starters and fillers, I change my words, I blink and screw up my face, I turn away.

I spent nearly 15 years as a solicitor. I had meetings, I used the phone, and I presented cases in court. Occasionally stammering helped, by stopping me saying the wrong thing, or giving me thinking time. But on the whole, stammering was a problem. People couldn't always understand what I was saying. I looked foolish – or at least I *felt* foolish, which is nearly the same thing. I faced prejudice from clients, from colleagues, and from prospective employers.

When I was 30, I took an intensive speech and language therapy course. That course, and top-up therapy since then, changed the way I felt about my stammer. I realized that the worst part was all of the non-stammer symptoms: avoiding words and situations; losing eye contact; using extra words and wrong words; and, worst of all, hating my stammer – and, as a result, hating myself. I learned how to deal with those symptoms. I can't be fluent, but I can be confident, be myself. I don't hate my stammer, and I don't hate myself.

I've come to realize that my stammer is part of what defines me, and that can be positive. When I phone a friend, I only have to say 'er', and they'll know who it is. If I'm reading to my children, it's fun for us all if I get stuck in the middle of a sentence. When I mention my stammer, people often share experiences or tell me about friends or relatives.

I've been to a national stammering conference. It was thrilling to be in a place full of stammerers. I felt like I'd met a long-lost family, I was coming home, I'd found a place where I belonged that I hadn't thought of before. All that I had to do to prove myself was to stammer. That's easy.

I gave up being a solicitor, for many reasons. Now I'm on a new journey. I'm training as a primary-school teacher. I like to explain my stammer to children. Sometimes it is new to them; sometimes they have heard a stammer, but not understood it. I love to see them try blocking for themselves, to watch them following my blocks or trying to guess what I'll say next. Many children have problems communicating, and my stammer can help me to help them, because children can relate to a person who is, like them, only human.

So I'm nearly friends with my stammer. Why 'nearly'? Because of my stammer, I will face self-doubt, prejudice and blocks. But my stammer will stay part of who I am, and it will help me to teach. We need to try to be friends.

Liz – age 47

I remember having a stammer from about the age of seven or eight. It just suddenly seemed to appear from nowhere. I remember a lot of good things about primary school, but always used to dread being asked my name. The same thing happened in secondary school, except now I avoided reading in class as much as possible; I was even asked by an English teacher if I found it difficult to read aloud. I said no, but what else was I going to say! It was too humiliating to admit that I was different from everyone else. Over the years, my stammer seemed to go away. But it had developed into what I now know to be a highly interiorized stammer. I seemed fluent, but I was pretty adept at avoiding saying certain words, sounds and situations. Nobody knew that I stammered, and as far as my family was concerned, I no longer had one (this is what I told them).

Work-wise, I worked in a lot of offices, doing IT (I could hide behind a computer screen). I did the odd presentation now and again, and said the odd word at work meetings, but I never felt comfortable. I felt frustrated that I had a lot to say and couldn't say it very well. I tried acting classes, sang in a choir (which helped), and even trained as a French teacher. I didn't stammer during my training, so what was that all about? But I did feel that I couldn't do teaching full time, just in case I stammered in front of the kids (or that's what I told myself).

Trying to hide my stammer was exhausting. I always had to think ahead and I'd had enough. I went along to an adult education centre that I'd been to for my acting/singing lessons and was recommended a few sessions with an individual speech and language therapist who pointed me in the direction of an evening class about interiorized stammering. I didn't want to admit that I still had a stammer, as I thought I'd 'cured' it – but who was I kidding! I learned a lot about the complex nature of stammering and about my own stammering, and it really helped me to be among other people with the same problem. I was introduced to a form of meditation which made me feel a lot calmer.

I found that I was saying words fluently that I hadn't said in years. I was even able to talk to friends about my stammer and found, to my amazement, that quite a few had guessed that I had a stammer, and they didn't care. I've always thought that I'd be rejected in some way if I 'confessed to the crime' of stammering. The difference now is that I accept my stammer; I'm still getting used to telling people about it and challenging other people's perceptions. And, I'm talking more fluently and calmly than before. I still have my bad days, but that's life.

Stammering is no longer something to be ashamed of.

Vicky – age 52

I'm 51 (52 this month) and started stammering when I was 19 years old, after having lived with my mother for that year. We had a very turbulent relationship and the first time I ever stammered was when a bloke was visiting me in my mother's flat. I knew she was listening to every word in the next room and it made me both angry and uptight. I was quite horrified to hear myself stammer. After he left, she asked me angrily how I could speak like that. A few weeks later, I stammered again and became aware that I could. It soon became a habit and, already shy and introverted, I withdrew even more. My mother would turn her back on me in the middle of a conversation as she hated to see and hear the stammer. For the next few years I stammered, but discussed it with nobody. I did a speech therapy course about four years later at the university where I was working. We worked on the continuous phonation technique which was very helpful, and by the end of the year I was up to a good speed (my previous speech was very, very fast). I'd always spoken fast, but, when stammering, wanted to get the words out even more quickly to prevent inflicting boredom!

After the therapy, I soon moved and lost the tenacity with which I'd practised the technique. I fell back into stammering, and did so for another 20 years! In the interim I'd become a passionate animal rights campaigner and vegan. About three years ago I attended a school speakers' workshop run by Viva!, which required volunteers to go into secondary schools and talk about meat-eating and how it affects our lives from various viewpoints: our health, the environment, and what it means for the animals themselves. The workshop was extremely inspiring. But how could I go into schools stammering away? I found a group therapy class for six months and it worked wonders. We had good fun, I was able to practise my school talk to many different people in and out of the group, and my confidence increased in leaps and bounds. It felt weird to be enjoying conversations, probably for the first time.

My first school rang me to do a talk before I'd finished the therapy and I panicked and said I wasn't ready. One of my speech and language therapy colleagues said I should just do it, and so I practised till I virtually knew it off by heart. The 20-minute talk went very well, the feedback was great, and I learnt something vital about myself. If it hadn't been for my stammer, I wouldn't have done the speech and language therapy courses – which gave me the confidence to go into schools and speak. I've done years of psychotherapy, read self-assertive books, etc., but it was the techniques learnt in group therapy that changed my life and enabled me to pursue my passion. Off to sleep now, as I have another talk first thing tomorrow morning!

Robert – age 55

I can remember as far back as when I was aged eight to ten and having the most blocking stammer. At the time I can remember feeling like a freak and being severely handicapped by it. My mother seemed to be in denial about it, despite the fact that her own mother and a cousin stammered. She would get very angry if I stammered near her. At school I found techniques to get round speaking. I would sit at the front of the class so that at least the classroom would not swivel round to see my contorting efforts.

I don't remember being teased by other children, but it must have happened. I would write down my destination when travelling on a bus or train, as well as writing down what I wanted in a shop or supermarket. I would get extremely anxious because of the pressure of needing to speak fluently. Invariably, the clerk would know about my stammer, and there would be people queuing up behind me. Singing was not a problem and it always surprised me. Why could I be fluent then, but not when speaking?

Using the telephone in one job I had as a cadet nurse became a nightmare as I was unable to call the ambulance to take out-patients home. It affected how well I could do my job. It was the same with other jobs over the next few years, and it was exacerbated if others were within earshot.

As an 18-year-old, I found a speech and language therapist in my local town. She was warm and encouraging and I began to learn that the more I relaxed and learned simple techniques, the more my fluency increased. This eased the most extreme aspects of the pattern, but the underlying habit remained well into my adult life.

I went on to train as a ballet dancer, which did not require me to use my voice – though there was one production where I was scripted and I was determined to see if I could speak on stage and on cue. I could in rehearsals, but they cut it all out prior to the first night due to time constraints (or that's what they told me!).

Although I am now largely, at 55 years old, a fluent speaker, and most colleagues and friends have no idea I have a speech problem, stammering is still an issue for me at times. In meetings I am not usually fluent. If I'm tired or nervous about what I have to say, there can be hesitancy. Even now, I am reduced to tears when I see productions that show a stammering young boy. On joining a stammerers' course some two to three years ago, I found myself feeling emotional about it and did not keep up contact with the other group members, though I did benefit from meeting them and having to stand up and speak in front of them. On the lighter side, as a younger man, I had a friend who also stammered – and the sight of the two of us together juddering through our communications did, at the time, fill me with ironic mirth.

David – age 67

I have been working hard on my speech for 22 years, having been spurred on by a particularly fluent episode. I saw no reason in principle why I should not be able to speak just as fluently in other situations. Since then I have been on most courses available – prolonged speech with soft contacts, block modification, passive air-flow, costal breathing, vocal fold management, also a smattering of NLP and Speaking Circles, together with lots of public speaking. To be honest, although I have derived some benefit from all my courses, none has been the definitive answer to what was a severe stammer.

Unfortunately speech and language therapists do not have all the answers. For most of the past 11 years I have been my own therapist. I have tried to get to the bottom of my problem. It has been a pick and mix of all the various techniques on offer, as well as incorporating my own ideas. The result is that I am vastly better and much more fluent than I ever was (and that's not just my opinion). What amazes me is that I am not totally fluent. I thought it would be easier than this, but I suppose, having learnt to stammer in the first place, I cannot simply unlearn at my age, just as I cannot unlearn to ride a bike. Techniques alone have not worked for me. Control of my feelings, my emotions, seems to be more important.

Do not give up. Do not be put off by those people who tell you there is no cure. You can improve enormously. You need to fly by the seat of your pants and instinctively feel what's good for you, what is doing you good. What's more, I'm still working on it, pushing forward the boundaries towards greater freedom of speech.

Paul – age 68

I attended school in rural Ireland in the 1940s and 1950s, and I was the only pupil who stammered. The teachers were unsympathetic, and I was often accused of 'putting it on' to avoid reading aloud or answering questions in class. I was frequently ridiculed by other pupils, and felt lonely, isolated and resentful. My parents took me to the family doctor, but he took the view that I would 'grow out of it' – he offered no practical help if I did not do so.

My stammer increased in severity and made my teenage years and twenties especially difficult. After I came to England I underwent a short course of speech and language therapy, but it was not effective. Avoiding words and situations became a way of life. On many occasions, I would steel myself to go into a feared situation only to back out at the last minute and then despise myself for doing so.

During my early thirties the severity of my stammer eased and I found that I could speak to people more freely and, more often than not, they would treat me with patience and courtesy. These new experiences encouraged me – my confidence improved greatly and I developed a more positive outlook on life.

I was not aware how much the understanding of stammering had advanced until I attended a course of speech and language therapy earlier this year. I found it insightful and helpful, and my fluency has improved. It was hard work, which is what I expected as I have stammered for so many years. I realize now that to retain the benefits of the course, I will have to practise the techniques I have learned for the rest of my life.

I hope that my experiences will give hope to older readers – it's never too late!

Appendix A

An example of a rating chart

Key

0 = no stammering
10 = the most you have heard your child stammer

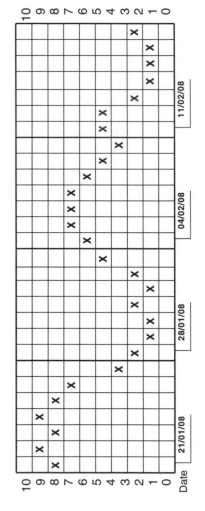

Figure A.1 A completed example of a rating chart

Appendix B
Blank rating chart

Key

0 = no stammering
10 = the most you have heard your child stammer

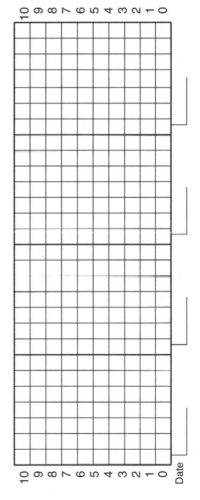

Figure B.1 A blank rating chart

Appendix C

Learning to speak at a slower rate with sufficient pauses

Reading practice

This programme is for anyone who is unable to obtain professional help and would like to work on slowing down and using pauses.
Remember:

- You are learning a new skill – the skill of speaking in an easier and more comfortable way.
- To be realistic – you cannot learn a new skill in a few hours or a few days.
- To be patient and go step by step – you are aiming to reduce rush and urgency.
- It will take time, but it will be worth it.
- Just as you cannot drive a car down a busy street after a couple of lessons or play football with professionals after a few training sessions, so you cannot gain control over your speech after a few hours of practice.

The usual progression when working on a speech technique is to start with:

Reading because the words are there for you, and you can concentrate on the technique.

Followed by:

1 *Monologue* – talking to yourself out loud for 1–2 minutes a few times a day. This is one step on from reading because you need to find your own words; however, there is no one to interrupt or hurry you.

2 *Monologue* – with just one person listening for 1–2 minutes. If there is someone to whom you can explain what you are doing – that is, talking out loud without interruption with one listener – then this is another step forward.

Finally:

Conversation is the last stage in terms of difficulty because you cannot control what the other person is going to say or when they are going to say it.

If you have a stopwatch, aim to start at approximately 40–60 words per minute (wpm). If you have no means of checking, think as follows:

40 wpm = very slow; 60 wpm = slow; 80 wpm = slow normal; 120–140 wpm = normal speaking rate

- Start by working at 40–60 wpm. Do not go for 60, 80 or 120 wpm until you feel confident using your slower, easier speech at this rate.
- Work for as long as you have time, but at least 10–20 minutes every day.

IMPORTANT: Remember to *pause*. In Chapter 10 we explained the crucial importance of pausing and, when working on your speech, it is essential that you introduce adequate pauses and practise with these pauses.

Practice passages

The reading passages below are supplied to give you an idea of the progression – starting with short phrases and increasing to longer passages. You may require more material, in which case you can count out the necessary number of words in a newspaper or magazine.

(1)

Many moons	Very soon	Now or never	Nearly there
New knives	You and me	All the same	This one
Why not	Very good	You and me	Go to school
In the oven	A red sky	Use the phone	How many more

(2)

We are near the sea
I wish it would rain
Are you sure about this?
No, we are not moving

Their house is far away
Where is the shop?
Where do you live?
The hills are alive

He is over there now
We will be landing soon
Some people are funny
Have you seen him?

(3)

I hope we can get to the match on time
I think it is time we started, don't you?
I wonder if it will be fine for the match
We were walking along that busy high street
Please get here in time for dinner
I hope you are feeling much better today
Yesterday at the zoo we saw this huge tiger
You will need a warm coat and hat tomorrow

(4)
20 words

When looking back, I was surprised to notice that not at any moment had I ever been at all frightened.

Once upon a time there was a little girl called Goldilocks who went alone for a walk in the woods.

When we started I found much pleasure in the cloudless sky, in the sunshine and the calm of green trees.

Talking in this way seems so easy and effortless that I will really try to remember how comfortable it feels.

(5)
40 words

Though houses in this country are often well built and fairly comfortable, there are more forms of dwelling to be found in other parts of the world. Houses can be made of ice, of straw, of mud and of leaves.

Like laughter, music is one of mankind's greatest gifts. Millions all over the world listen to popular music played on the radio, television and iPods. A smaller audience listens regularly to other kinds of music such as classical or jazz.

(6)
60 words

Today no opportunities for adventure remain. There are no lands still unexplored, no dark secret interiors tempt the explorer with the possibility of wonderful discoveries. All seas are known and charted, and the days of risky sail are gone as heavy iron ships sail swiftly across the waves. The adventurous still look for thrills and excitement in far away places.

(7)
Longer passage

At first glance this may seem a simple case for you to decide, but it is not as simple as it seems. A quantity of evidence has been produced which throws suspicion on this young man. This evidence includes that he had shown particular interest in this computer, which he admitted that he could not afford; he was in the shop at or about the time that the computer was stolen, and the shop was crowded at the time so that he could, you may think, have taken the computer away unobserved. The item was later found by the police in his room. No one, however, saw him take the computer and the defence has shown that at least fifty other people had the same opportunity of taking it. The prisoner has told you in the witness box that he bought the computer cheaply from this young man called 'Shorty'. You might consider this mysterious person an invention of the prisoner were it not for the fact that his existence has been proved by the evidence of the leader of the youth club.

Guidelines for practising

- Consider your practice on three different levels.
- All levels are to be practised every day once the required stage has been reached, i.e. do not stop practising level 1 once you start level 2.
- Short frequent practice sessions are better than one long session every few days.

LEVEL 1 – Practising while alone

Sometimes people who stammer say that it is a waste of time practising reading alone as they do not stammer while reading on their own. Remember: the aim of the technique is not to see how often you can stammer, but to build on increasing fluency, and the feeling of fluency until this becomes automatic.

- Practise reading and talking when on your own for a short time every day.
- Work at various speeds – not necessarily counting wpm, but going very slowly, slowly and at an average rate.
- If possible, occasionally use a recording device to check your work.
- Think of Level 1 practice like training for a particular sport when you

need to increase your fitness and stamina quite slowly, over a period of time, using exercises some of which are for practice purposes only. You are now in training to gain control over your speech.

LEVEL 2 – Practising with one close friend/relative

At this level of practice you are transferring your technique from working by yourself into a conversation with one other person.

- Explain to the other person what you are doing.
- Explain why you are practising this new way of talking (explanation is important so that your listener understands what is going on and is not confused by the change in your speech).
- Your friend should speak in his or her usual way, but you should start at approximately 60 wpm and move slowly to 80 wpm.
- Do not go for a marathon – just aim for short conversations.
- Gradually increase the length of time that you are speaking in this way.

LEVEL 3 – Practising in everyday life

Your ultimate aim is to use this easier way of speaking at a normal speaking rate in your everyday life.

- People are far too busy to analyse your speech and, although you may feel strange at first, others may be unaware or uninterested in *how* you speak because they are more interested in *what* you are saying.
- You do not always need to be fluent – just concentrate on one conversation at a time.
- You are bound to stammer occasionally, but this does not mean that you are back at square one or that you have failed. Whatever activity we are engaged in, no one gets it right all the time – it is how you react when you stammer that is important. Think of your hierarchy, how far have you come from where you started? Instead of being angry with yourself, you should be proud that you have taken the time and energy to do this work on your speech.

Audio materials to aid practice

New audio and visual materials are constantly being developed, and it is worth regularly checking the websites of stammering associations to see if any have been released that you may find useful.

Appendix D
Breathing exercises

Most breathing exercises can be performed either in the sitting position, or lying on the floor. If sitting, make sure you are in a comfortable position with your back erect but not rigid; if lying on the floor, put a small pillow under your neck to avoid strain.

Start by working for five minutes and then increase the time slowly. If you feel dizzy, light-headed or faint, stop immediately and rest.

The exercises should always be done in a calm and unhurried manner so that the muscles are able to expand and contract without strain. Do not push yourself or your breath – gently does it!

Guidelines for breathing exercises:

- Balance exercise with rest. If you feel tired, rest and try again. If you feel very tired, stop and start again the next day.
- Wait at least one hour after eating before beginning an exercise.
- If you've been away from these exercises for several days, start up slowly and gradually return to your regular routine.

Breathing to expand your lung capacity

This exercise is best done lying down, but if that is difficult, it is possible to do it in a sitting position:

- Lie down and put your hands, palms downwards, on your stomach just under the rib cage, and with the middle fingers barely touching.
- Take a deep breath and, as you breathe in, the stomach will expand slightly and the fingertips will separate.
- Breathe out and, as you breathe out, gently push the stomach and diaphragm inwards.
- Do this for 3–5 minutes.

Breathing for vocal fold vibration

Do the same breathing pattern as for the previous exercise but, as you breathe out, close your lips and make a humming sound. Hold this for as long as you can, but stop when the sound becomes weak. Make sure you can feel the vibration forward in the mouth on your lips, and not right back in your throat.

Do this for 3–5 minutes.

Breathing to increase energy

This is a noisy breathing exercise. Inhale and exhale rapidly through your nose. Breathe in and out as quickly as possible. Keep the mouth closed, but make sure that the area round the mouth, neck and shoulders is relaxed.

To start, do three in and out breaths (one cycle), and then breathe normally for a moment. This is a powerful exercise ensuring quick movements of the diaphragm, so do not do more than three cycles when starting. Increase very slowly, and do not exceed six cycles at a time.

Breathing for relaxation

You can do this exercise in almost any position, but it might be easiest to start off with sitting:

- Put the tip of your tongue against the ridge just behind your top teeth and keep your tongue there throughout the exercise. You can purse your lips slightly if you find that more comfortable.
- Breathe out through your mouth, making a 'rushing' sound.
- Shut your mouth and breathe in silently through your nose to a count of four.
- Hold your breath to a count of four. As you become more experienced, you can gradually increase this to a count of five, then six, and finally seven.
- Breathe out, making a rushing sound to a count of four. Gradually increase this to a count of five, then six, and finally seven.
- The inhaling phase should remain at a count of four, while the other phases are gradually increased.
- Do this exercise 3–4 times only.

Vocal cord or vocal fold vibration

This is an expanded exercise started in Chapter 11. It may be easier if you close your eyes.

- Breathe in and, as you breathe out, make a gentle humming sound, like mmmmmmmm. Try to feel the vibration of your vocal cords. It may help to put your hand on the front of your throat at about the level of your Adam's apple. It may be beneficial to close your eyes.

- Repeat this five times and check that your voice is forward in the mouth so that you can feel a slight tingle or vibration on your lips.
- Breathe out, gently breathe in and, on the outgoing breath, keep the vibration going on eeeeeeeeee. Repeat three times.
- Then do as above, but using ooooooooo. Repeat three times.
- Repeat with 'oh'.
- Do this exercise for 5 minutes, always checking that you are aware of the vibration in your throat. Continue until you feel that you have increased your awareness of vocal cord movement.
- Add some one-syllable words (keeping the same easy pattern of vibration in your throat) – mmmmy; mmmore; mmmman; wwww-wwhy; wwwwhen; fffffine; fffffun; fffffffor; sssssee; ssssssun; sssssssay; rrrrrrred; rrrrrrrun; rrrrrrroad; you can add some words of your own. Note that some of the words start with a voiced sound and others with one that is voiceless. Feel the difference.
- If you are secure with the work so far, move on. Stay at the stage where you are comfortable and experience vibration, and do not move on to the next stage until you are ready. There is no rush with this work.
- Now *speak* the one-syllable words with the same vibration in your throat, and with the same easy start that you used when you were practising the previous exercises. It is useful to elongate the first sound very slightly at this stage – my, more, man, why, when, fine, fun, sun, look, low, line, so, see, say, road, red, run. Add some one-syllable words of your own. Make sure you are speaking, and not chanting.
- Progress to two words – each word of one syllable: why here?; just now; see them; go there; stand up; show over; take care; sit down; big car; good-bye; over here; read this; ten times; for now. You might want to add combinations of one-syllable words of your own.

When you have done these exercises regularly, and for a considerable length of time, you will have become more aware of vocal cord vibration. You can now begin to experiment with making sure that you bring this vibration, or voice, into sounds as you speak – this is especially important at the beginning of words. When talking, as you breathe out, focus on using the same gentle onset to the voice that you have practised in this exercise, so that you reduce any tendency to hurry or to increase tension in the cords.

Appendix E
Negative thoughts

Negative thoughts are unhelpful and tend to cluster under a number of headings. Here are some of them:

- Thinking in extremes – this is when there are no grey areas. Everything is either absolutely perfect or a terrible disaster.
- 'Should', 'ought to', 'must' and 'have to' are words which, when used carelessly, can presume standards and rules that do not actually exist. They imply dire consequences for not obeying and may create anxiety and guilt – for example, by law you 'should' obey a red traffic light. Is it equally true that 'I should have done better at this job' or 'I must not stammer'? Who says?
- Negative labels – these are the words that are used to make you lose confidence and lower both your own self-esteem and that of others. Words like 'stupid', 'lazy', 'fat' and 'boring' are seriously negative. Thinking about yourself (or other people) with these word labels can make you believe that this is part of your identity, and so you can begin to be highly critical of yourself. This is guaranteed to lower your feelings of self-esteem and confidence.
- Jumping to conclusions. You can jump to conclusions in two ways:

1 By 'mind reading'. This is when you decide that you know that your boss is angry with you, your neighbour does not like you, or that your friend is embarrassed by your stammer. How do you know this? What evidence do you have?
2 By expecting the worst will happen, again without evidence: 'What if I mess up the interview?' or 'What if no one likes me?' Expecting the worst creates anxiety, and so affects your performance and stops you from doing your best.

- Blaming yourself – you tend to blame yourself for things for which you were either not responsible, or only partly responsible. You overlook others who were involved and who must also be accountable.

Exercise 1

Photocopy Form 1 (Figure E.1), or use the form given below. Fill it in by writing down events as soon after they occur as possible; we have given one example on the form. Do this for one week as it will help you to become aware of what you are doing and how you think and feel.

Situation Day Approx. time	How did you feel?	What were your thoughts?	On a scale of 1–10 how negative were the thoughts?
Monday 10.10 a.m. I stammered a lot on the phone. Shilpa noticed and commented	Embarrassed Ashamed Stupid	Shilpa thinks I'm no good at this job. I'll have problems next time the phone rings	8 and they lasted on and off for most of the morning

Figure E.1   Form 1

After doing this for a week, you will be ready to take a further step and use Form 2 (Figure E.2) to help you record how realistic your thoughts are when expressed as a percentage. As near as possible to the time of the event, write down how true you believed these thoughts were at the moment when you felt really negative. See Form 2 for an example.

Situation Day Approx. time	How did you feel?	What were your thoughts?	How negative were the thoughts? Was there anything positive in that situation?	How true do you think these thoughts are? 100% true? 75% true? 50% true? 30%? Not true at all?
Wednesday 7.50 a.m. Buying a ticket to Waterloo. Long queue. Bad stammer Stuck on 'w'	Scared Ashamed Angry with myself	Why me? I should have been able to say it. I think I was stuck for ages.	Very negative Positive: I went for it rather than avoid it and I got there in the end, and I got my ticket	About 40% true

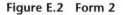

Figure E.2   Form 2

Third week – what have you discovered in the first two weeks?

> *I have discovered . . .*

Exercise 2

Now put an elastic band round your wrist to act as a reminder. Select one that is comfortable for you and, when you become aware of a negative thought, touch the elastic band and STOP. Don't allow yourself to pursue that thought, but rather begin to think what you could tell yourself that would be true at this time, and more helpful and positive. It must be a thought that is honest because otherwise you will not believe it, so that telling yourself 'nobody is listening to my conversation' or 'I won't stammer' or 'I don't care if I stammer' may not be the truth for you. It is jumping straight from negative to positive without any in-between stages.

- Ask yourself, 'Is what I am telling myself realistic or is it a half truth, illogical or a distortion of reality?' For example, 'I know that when I get to the ticket office tomorrow morning, I won't be able to say a word' (expecting the worst/thinking in extremes/being unrealistic). You might agree that this is a half-truth (you may well have some difficulty asking for your ticket, but it is also a distortion of reality because you *will* be able to say 'a word'). Apart from that, are you a fortune-teller? How is it that you can predict the future with such accuracy? You cannot know for sure what will happen tomorrow.

Keep repeating your exercise in positive self-talk several times per day, and you will be surprised how this will gradually become automatic and increase your confidence and self-esteem.

You were not born with all the thoughts that you have now. These thoughts have grown and multiplied over the years as you began to worry about your stammer. They are *your* thoughts. *You* can change them with a little hard work.

Exercise 3

Complete this exercise as soon as possible after you have done something that caused you to employ negative self-talk. Write down the answer to each of the following questions. Put the paper away and look at it again the next day. Any new thoughts?

What happened during the event?

What did I tell myself about it?

What effect did my self-talk have on the situation?

Under similar circumstances, how could I alter my self-talk in the future?

How might a change of self-talk affect the situation?

Appendix F
Avoidance reduction

Monitoring

Monitoring or checking what you are doing is central to this approach. If you really monitor well, you will automatically begin to drop many of your secondary behaviours or strategies. You can make quicker progress by alert monitoring than by constantly trying to stop your acquired stammering behaviours.

Suggested exercise:
When you are in a situation and find yourself using avoidances, observe exactly the series of things that you do before, during and after the stammer. It is not enough to think 'I stammered'; you need to observe more precisely.

Sean's observation read like this: 'I went to meet Mick after work and found that he had brought his girlfriend along. I find her difficult to talk to. I knew I was going to stammer, but decided to use this situation as an open stammering opportunity. I noticed that I was breathing quite quickly. I definitely looked away before starting to speak and, for what seemed ages but was probably only a second, my cords closed and I didn't make a sound. Unfortunately, I pushed the word out when I know I could have just paused and eased through it; I think my habit of pushing is so strong that I forget to pause and ease into the word. Surprisingly, I didn't feel too bad.'

You will progress much further and speak more easily if you keep seeking out feared words and situations instead of just letting them happen to you. You cannot stand still – so you are either advancing further into open stammering or moving back into avoidance.

Suggested exercise:
Find one situation, or one word every day, for the specific purpose of working on open stammering. You can choose a familiar situation, a new situation or a word that you would normally avoid. Monitor well and keep eye contact. Write down what happened – With whom? What did you do? How did you feel?

Counting successes and failures

In open stammering, you can count the following as successes:

- Stammer with good eye contact.
- Go out of your way to find a situation especially for your speech.
- Use no substitutions, postponers or starters.
- Complete any feared word that you start.
- Monitor well – observe exactly what you do when you stammer.
- Talk to someone about your stammer.
- Think: 'I stammer – so what?'

Count it as a failure if you:

- substitute, postpone or use a starter;
- look away during a block;
- go back and 'take a run' at a feared word;
- try to talk fluently whatever the cost;
- do not make a sound when you block;
- cover up your stammer by whatever means.

	Establish eye contact before speaking	Keep eye contact while stammering	Use a feared word	Complete a feared word when starting to stammer	Talk to someone about your stammer	Pick one feared situation and do it in spite of the fear
Monday						
Tuesday						
Wednesday						
Thursday						
Friday						
Saturday						
Sunday						

Figure F.1   Form 3

You might like to use a timetable to check your progress. See Form 3 (Figure F.1). Decide how many of the columns you are ready to tackle and set yourself a realistic goal.

Talking about your stammer

For many people, this is hard, but it is worth remembering that you are reading this chapter because you feel uncomfortable speaking at certain times, or even most of the time. You have tried to hide and avoid your stammer as best you can for much of your adult life and yet you are still uncomfortable. Why? Only you can answer that question. For many, it is because avoidance is tiring, saps your energy and, worst of all, is not honest – you cannot be yourself while pretending to be fluent.

When you reach the stage of being able to talk about your stammer openly and easily, if this is appropriate to the situation, then you will know that fluency achieved by hiding and pretending increases your fear of stammering, and being open and honest reduces fear and tension.

Suggested exercise:
Try to talk about your stammer to one (easy) person, but make sure you are using the same terms. Some people believe that there is a difference between stammering and stuttering – and consider that stuttering is more serious. Others, however, believe just the opposite.

- You will need to open the conversation.
- Bear in mind that the other person can be quite unsure what to say, so be prepared to keep the conversation going.
- 'What do you think about my stammer?' is not a helpful question, partly because the person may answer 'I don't think about it at all' or have no response at all because the question has put them on the spot.
- More helpful, you could try saying something about yourself, such as, 'I've always avoided talking about my stammer, but I'd really like to tell you what I am practising at the moment.' It is true to say that 80–90 per cent of our clients who have started to talk about their speech have been surprised by the results. This is often such a huge step for people who stammer that they are amazed at their feeling of great freedom and strength by doing this, and at the casual response of the listener.

Useful addresses

The British Stammering Association
15 Old Ford Road
London E2 9PJ
Tel.: 020 8983 1003
Helpline: 0845 603 2001
Website: www.stammering.org

Stammering or Stuttering Associations throughout the world are too numerous to list here. The best way to find an organization in the country where you live is to go to <http://www.mnsu.edu/comdis/kuster/support.html>.

Stuttering Foundation of America
3100 Walnut Grove, Suite 603
P.O. Box 11749
Memphis
TN 38111-0749
USA
Website: www.stutteringhelp.org

www.stuttersfa.org

The Stuttering Home Page
Minnesota State University
Mankato
MN 56001
USA
Website: www.stutteringhomepage.org

National Stuttering Association
119 West 40th Street, 14th Floor
New York
NY 10018
USA
Website: www.nsastutter.org

Friends (National Association of Young People Who Stutter)
Website: www.friendswhostutter.org

Employment issues and stammering
Website: www.stammeringlaw.org.uk

Royal College of Speech and Language Therapists
2 White Hart Yard
London SE1 1NX
Tel.: 020 7378 1299
Website: www.rcslt.org

City Literary University (City Lit) Speech Therapy Team
Keeley Street
London WC2B 4BA
Tel.: 020 7492 2578/9
Website: www.citylit.ac.uk/cou_sub_st.php
Email: speechtherapy@citylit.ac.uk

Michael Palin Centre for Stammering Children
Finsbury Health Centre
Pine Street
London EC1R 0LP
Tel.: 020 7530 4238
Website: www.stammeringcentre.org

Association of Speech and Language Therapists in Independent Practice
Coleheath Bottom
Speen
Princes Risborough
Bucks HP27 0SZ
Tel.: 01494 488306
Website: www.helpwithtalking.com

ChildLine (a service of the NSPCC)
Weston House
42 Curtain Road
London EC2A 3NH
Tel.: 0800 1111
Website: www.childline.org.uk

Parentline Plus
520 Highgate Studios
53–79 Highgate Road
Kentish Town
London NW5 1TL
Tel.: 0808 800 2222
Website: www.parentlineplus.org.uk

Kidscape
2 Grosvenor Gardens
London SW1W 0DH
Tel.: 08451 205 204
Website: www.kidscape.org.uk

Stammering and the Disability Discrimination Act (1995)
Website: www.stammeringlaw.org.uk

Equality and Human Rights Commission
Website: www.equalityhumanrights.com

British Association for Counselling and Psychotherapy (BACP)
BACP House
15 St John's Business Park
Lutterworth
Leics. LE17 4HB
Tel.: 0870 443 5252
Website: www.bacp.co.uk

British Society of Clinical Hypnosis
125 Queensgate
Bridlington
East Yorkshire YO16 7JQ
Tel.: 01262 403103
Website: www.bsch.org.uk

National Register of Hypnotherapists and Psychotherapists (NRHP)
Suite B, 12 Cross Street
Nelson
Lancashire BB9 7EN
Tel.: 01282 716839
Website: www.nrhp.co.uk

Neuro-Linguistic Programming and Stammering
Dr Mike Jones can provide information on this method.
Email: mike.reprogram@connectfree.co.uk
You can also go to the website <www.stammering.org> and search on 'NLP' or 'Mike Jones'.

Personal Construct Psychology
Peggy Dalton
20 Cleveland Avenue
London W4 1SN
Tel.: 020 8994 7959
Website: www.pcpet.org.uk
Email: daltonpcp@aol.com

Peggy Dalton can provide information about this field of psychology and its help with stammering.

The Association of Speakers Clubs
Website: www.the-asc.org.uk

Toastmasters International
Website: www.toastmasters.org

Notes

1 Adapted from an analogy formulated by the late Dr Joseph Sheehan (formerly Professor of Psychology, University of California).
2 Gregory's headings were 'Stutter more Fluently' and 'Speak more Fluently'. The former heading causes some confusion and is now often referred to as 'Stutter more Easily' or 'Stammer more Easily'.

Further reading

There is a huge choice of books, videos, CDs and DVDs on the subjects listed below. These are available through bookshops, libraries, health stores, the British Stammering Association, and the internet.

We make no claim that the titles listed here are preferable to other titles, but offer them in the hope that they will lead you to the material that you require.

Stammering – general

Emerick, L. (ed.), *Advice To Those Who Stutter*. Speech Foundation of America, Memphis, 1998.

Murray, F., *Stutterer's Story*. Speech Foundation of America, Memphis, 1980.

Tunbridge, N., *The Stutterer's Survival Guide*. Addison-Wesley, New York, 1994.

For teachers

Rustin, L., Cook, F., Botterill, W., Hughes, C. and Kelman, E., *Stammering: A Practical Guide for Teachers and Other Professionals*. David Fulton Publishers, London, 2001.

For parents

Faber, A. and Mazlish, E., *How to Talk so Kids will Listen and Listen so Kids will Talk*. Avon Books, New York, 1980.

Golden, B., *Healthy Anger – How to Help Children and Teens Manage Their Anger*. Oxford University Press, Oxford, 2006.

Guitar, B., Guitar, C. and Fraser, J., *Stuttering and the Preschool Child: Help for Families*. Videotape. Stuttering Foundation of America, Memphis, 2000.

Social skills, assertiveness and anger management

Braiker, H., *The Disease To Please*. McGraw-Hill, New York, 2002.

Dryden, W. and Constantinou, D., *Assertiveness: Step by Step*. Sheldon Press, London, 2005.

Elman, N. M. and Kennedy-Moore, E., *The Unwritten Rules of Friendship*. Little, Brown, New York, 2003. (Social skills for children)

Favaro, P., *Anger Management*. Pentagon Press, Warwick, 2005.

Gabor, D., *How to Start a Conversation and Make Friends*. Sheldon Press, London, 1983.

Hartley, M., *The Assertiveness Handbook*. Sheldon Press, London, 2006.

Bullying

Cohen-Posey, K., *How to Handle Bullies, Teasers and Other Meanies*. Rainbow Books, USA, 1995.

Elliot, M., *The Willow Street Kids Beat the Bullies*. Macmillan Children's Books, London, 1986.

Lawson, S., *Helping Children Cope with Bullying*. Sheldon Press, London, 1994.

Yaruss, J. S., Murphy, B., Quesal, R. W. and Rearden, N. A., *Bullying and Teasing – Helping Children Who Stutter: A Manual for Speech-Language Pathologists, Teachers, Administrators, and Children Who Stutter*. National Stuttering Association, New York, 2004.

Self-esteem, confidence and stress

Fennell, M., *Overcoming Low Self-Esteem – A Self-Help Guide Using Cognitive Behavioural Techniques*. Arrow Books, London, 1991.

Jeffers, S., *Feel the Fear and Do It Anyway – How to Turn Your Fear and Indecision Into Confidence and Action*. Ballantine Books, London, 2006.

McCracken, A., *The Stress Gremlins*. ARIMA Publishing, Suffolk, 2005.

Relaxation and meditation

Bodian, S. and Ornish, D., *Meditation for Dummies*. For Dummies, Yorkshire, 2006.

Davis, M., Eshelman, E. and McKay, M., *The Relaxation and Stress Reduction Workbook*. New Harbinger Publications, Oakland, CA, 2000.

Kabat-Zinn, J., *Wherever You Go, There You Are – Mindfulness Meditation in Everyday Life*. Hyperion Books, New York, 1994.

Zeer, D., *Office Yoga – Simple Stretches for Busy People*. Chronicle Books, Yorkshire, 2000.

Counselling

Andreas, S., *NLP: The New Technology*. HarperCollins, USA, 1996.

Bodenhamer, B., *Mastering Blocking and Stuttering*. Crown House Publishing, Carmarthen, 2004.

Dryden, W. and Feltham, C., *Counselling and Psychotherapy – A Consumer's Guide*. Sheldon Press, London, 1995.

Sanders, P., *First Steps in Counselling*. PCCS books, Ross-on-Wye, 2002.

Index